C000008327

The Brightness Of Healing

– ELSPETH SCOTT –

An environmentally friendly book printed and bound in England by
www.printondemand-worldwide.com

Mixed Sources
Product group from well-managed
forests, and other controlled sources
www.fsc.org Cert no. TT-COC-002641
© 1996 Forest Stewardship Council

PEFC Certified

This product is
from sustainably
managed forests
and controlled
sources

www.pefc.org

PEFC/16-33-415

This book is made entirely of chain-of-custody materials

i

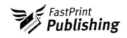

www.fast-print.net/store.php

The Brightness Of Healing

Copyright © Elspeth Scott 2011

Edited by Emma Tuck

DISCLAIMER

The information in this book is made available on the understanding that the author is providing material based on her own personal approaches and experiences. The text does not cover all possible uses, actions, precautions and side effects. Interactions and liability for individual actions or omissions based on the contents of this book is expressly disclaimed.

ISBN 978-178035-235-0

First published 2011 by
FASTPRINT PUBLISHING
Peterborough, England.

Thank you to all those who have encouraged me in writing this book, especially my friend Lucy.

In memory of my mother.

Contents

Preface

Health is not simply a matter of absence of illness. Health means constant challenge. Constant creativity. A prolific life always moving forward, opening up fresh new vistas – that is a life of true health. An unbeatable spirit is what supplies the power to keep pressing ahead. [1]

It is now over ten years since I first developed a painful bladder illness following years of cystitis attacks leading to repeated courses of antibiotics. I had also suffered with urethritis (pain and irritation in the urethra) for six years, together with a myriad of other chronic symptoms such as intestinal problems, sore throats, bloating and headaches – all indications of a compromised immune system struggling to cope. Whilst these types of symptoms are relatively common, they were easier to ignore than the damage that was being caused to my bladder.

Whatever I ate or drank made the relentless pain in my bladder worse but being undiagnosed or misdiagnosed was, and perhaps still is, a familiar problem for those suffering from interstitial cystitis. Had I foreseen the drastic consequences of my body's immune system becoming steadily weakened and out of balance, and the negative impact this would have on my life, I would have taken action sooner to enable my own recovery.

After exploring many avenues and using a combination of alternative treatments and approaches, my health gradually began to improve. When I attended my annual hospital appointment about six and a half years later and informed the consultant that I had recovered, his response was that I had gone into remission. To this date I have never returned to the situation that I was in and, although I try to lead a much healthier lifestyle now, I am able to eat and drink whatever I like.

At the onset of interstitial cystitis (also known as bladder pain syndrome), my main wish was to be told that at least one person had managed to fully recover; the illness has a continuum of stages and I know that there are those who are further down the line with this condition. It took me a number of years to make any progress. It felt as if I was trying to unravel a huge and complicated knot – but perhaps there was a simpler answer if only I could find it.

This book gives a personal approach to overcoming a problem that many people suffer from, often over many years. I live in an area where I can access treatment and health food shops selling good quality supplements, but I am aware that these are not always available. However, it has now become much easier to buy products via the internet. My aim is to offer encouragement and information to enable others to help themselves get better. It outlines the remedies, treatments and changes to lifestyle that I undertook to aid my recovery from a painful bladder, together with ways to maintain a healthy immune system.

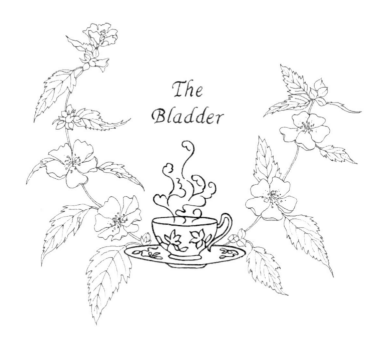

The Bladder

In biological terms the bladder is often described as a hollow organ consisting of muscle with an inner lining which is used to store urine until it is released from the body. I have only found one reference to the fact that the bladder is one of the most sensitive organs. This is because the layers of tissue inside the bladder have a high supply of nerves to enable it to perform its function. The bladder has three layers: an outer layer of soft connective tissue; a muscle coat where the nerves are carried; and an inner layer of mucous membrane. The sensation that gives us the signal to want to empty our bladder is caused by chemicals in the urine leaking across the inner membrane as it gradually becomes stretched. The nerves are then triggered to respond.

The inner layers of the bladder are made up of delicate tissues. These can become damaged or eroded when infections occur because bacteria secrete enzymes which enable them to stick to the bladder wall. The bacteria then begin to colonise, causing further infection. When the bladder is full the walls are stretched, but otherwise the inner mucous membrane lies in folds – which is why one is required to drink so much water before having a cystoscopy (an internal examination of the bladder using a cystoscope). Urine is an acidic substance that can irritate already inflamed tissues causing additional pain, so the healing of scar tissue within the bladder can be a lengthy and complicated process.

The impact of an inflamed or damaged bladder on sufferers, in terms of pain or lifestyle restrictions, can be very hard to talk about and is rarely openly discussed. The varying types of reaction – from stabbing or burning pains to spasm of the bladder muscle – is also evidence of the degree of sensitivity of this organ. However, the range and unpredictability of symptoms can be quite alarming.

Women are much more commonly affected by cystitis than men due to their shorter urethra which makes the bladder more susceptible to infection from unfriendly bacteria. Around 50% of women will require treatment for a urinary tract infection during their lifetime.[2]

In Traditional Chinese Medicine the bladder is an aspect of the water element and is associated with the emotion of fear. Hence, when a person becomes fearful or anxious they may need to urinate more frequently, or in situations of extreme fear temporary loss of bladder control can occur. The qualities of the bladder are connected with courage and the ability to move forward in life.

The bladder is situated at the base of the abdomen and is described as being within the realm of the sacral chakra (and also the base chakra). There are seven major chakras, or energy centres, in the body and each one regulates the organs found in its particular area. The sacral chakra, located below the naval, is connected with creativity and the balance between our inner and outer selves. Although it is governed by the moon it is also related to the water element, and therefore affects our emotional stability. Its colour is orange. The base chakra, situated at the bottom of the spine, is the red coloured root of the lotus and is connected with survival and security as well being the source of courage, strength, willpower and energy.

The location of the bladder and urethra, and their connection via the nervous system to the sexual organs in women (and the rectum in men), undoubtedly makes pain in this area all the more significant because of the impact this can have on an emotional as well as a physical level.

Bacterial Cystitis versus Interstitial Cystitis

'Cyst' derives from the Greek *kustis*, which means bladder or sac and the suffix 'itis' denotes disease or inflammation. 'Interstitial' describes the way the infection takes root in or between small areas of organ tissue.

When I first developed the constant burning symptoms in my bladder I discovered the book *You Don't Have to Live with Cystitis* by Larrian Gillespie in my local library. She describes interstitial cystitis as 'one of the least understood and most under-diagnosed diseases in modern urology'.[3]

Having suffered from repeated cystitis attacks and many years of urethritis (a common precursor to interstitial cystitis) I knew that what I was experiencing was different to a normal bladder infection. For example, one of the hallmarks of interstitial cystitis is the pain before and after voiding but not during; with a typical cystitis infection the pain occurs during urination. The pain of interstitial cystitis is continuous. Unlike common cystitis no bacteria are found to be present in a urine test, although a negative culture cannot rule out all types of infection.

With interstitial cystitis it is thought that damage has been caused to the GAG (glycosaminoglycan) layer in the bladder, which normally protects against the acids and toxins in urine, causing it to become leaky. As a result, the pH of the urine can become more alkaline.

The burning pain of interstitial cystitis is caused by inflammation of the interstice (or interstitium) – the area between the bladder lining and muscle. Furthermore, the exposed nerves in the damaged tissue are unable to heal, as with normal scar tissue, because they are continually coming into contact with urine due to a defective GAG layer. The inflammation can lead to scarring and stiffening of the bladder, decreased bladder capacity, pinpoint bleeding (glomerulations) and, in some cases, the formation of ulcers on the bladder wall.

Research suggests that interstitial cystitis may be an autoimmune disease, which means that the body's immune system has become confused and turned on itself, attacking its own tissue.

Painful intercourse can also be caused by interstitial cystitis because chemicals (the neurotransmitters acetylcholine, morepinephrine, and serotonin) are carried along nerves which travel from the brain to the heart, gut, bladder, urethra and then into the clitoris. The nerves run between the base of the bladder and the vagina, so the burning pain is intensified as these nerves are stimulated.

Dr Gillespie talks about 'agents' that serve as promoters of interstitial cystitis and states that environmental factors can play an important role in the formation of this illness. She says that the disease process can begin when presensitised people come into contact with one or more environmental factors. The onset can be quite sudden for some people, but slow for others.[4]

Although I was not fully aware of the problem, I had become sensitive to chemicals including those in some everyday products such as antibacterial soaps, but it was following exposure to chemicals in the form of pesticides that the onset of the illness properly began. I had known that something was wrong as my urine had become very cloudy (a sign of possible infection in the bladder), I was finding it hard to stay awake as my energy levels had dropped dramatically and I developed a pain that felt different to my usual attacks of cystitis. I described this feeling to my doctor who prescribed antibiotics, which only made the pain in my bladder worse. Links have been made between incidences of bladder pain, as well as other problems, due to exposure to harmful chemicals and pesticides.[5]

Dr Gillespie identifies three antibiotics that link her interstitial cystitis patients: nitrofurantoin, tetracycline and erythromycin.[6] I had taken tetracycline for a considerable time to treat skin problems and I had also taken nitrofurantoin for bladder infections. I subsequently read a feature in the health section of *The Sunday Times Style* magazine in which the practitioner was asked about the effects of long-term antibiotics to treat a skin problem by a mother concerned about her daughter's bloating and constipation. She refers to advice from an alternative skin specialist who says that antibiotic treatment is likely to have affected the kidney, bladder and lymphatic functioning and therefore resulted in urinary infections. As a treatment she recommended cranberry tablets, Citricidal (see Chapter 2) and also blue-green algae (see Chapter 5).[7]

Problems occur when antibiotics are prescribed for a bladder infection without first identifying the particular bacteria, combined with an already weak and sensitive system. Antibiotics can treat a true attack of bacterial cystitis as they will target the microorganisms, although it is important to replenish the good bacteria in the body's system by taking probiotics (see Chapter 4). If there are symptoms of a bladder infection and no bacteria are found, the problem could be due to a fungal infection, in which case antibiotics may make this worse.

During my time of experiencing the burning within my bladder I did not suffer from common cystitis attacks, although I have read of others who experience both at the same time. Bacteria do not thrive well in either very acid or alkaline environments, which is why it can help to take bicarbonate of soda to make the urine more alkaline, although this is not recommended on a regular basis. Obviously, the aim is to heal the bladder in order to prevent the pain from occurring.

The Immune System

Our immune system provides the body with self-protection from invading organisms such as bacteria, viruses, fungi and any other harmful substances. We have an *innate* immunity that we are born with and also an *adaptive* or *acquired* immunity whereby the body will respond specifically to fight off an invading microorganism.

The lymphatic system is a second circulatory system to our blood system and one of its main functions is to manufacture white blood cells which destroy harmful bacteria. In Chinese Traditional Medicine there is also the meridian system based on an ancient philosophy of energy channels within our bodies. There are twelve major organ meridians, and signals or imbalances linked to these can point to ill health before a disease manifests.

Enzymes play a very crucial role in our bodies by enabling chemical reactions to take place and allowing vitamins, minerals and hormones to do their work. These proteins are also responsible for strengthening the immune system, breaking down and eliminating toxins, cleansing the blood and facilitating repair and healing processes within the body. An example of an enzyme deficiency is lactose intolerance, in which the lactase enzyme needed to break down lactose, the main sugar found in milk and other dairy products, is lacking.

Nowadays our bodies have to deal with an increasing number of harmful contaminants and pollutants in our environment and through the things that we consume in our diets, including hidden antibiotics in meat, pesticide residues in foods and chemical residues in our drinking water (see Chapter 7). There is also evidence of a strong link between our emotional state and our immune system – its abilities can be impaired due to stress and trauma in our lives.

In a healthy body the urethra (and the intestines) contain friendly bacteria that guard against bladder infections as well as being protected by mucus. These bacteria can be destroyed through the use of antibiotics which indiscriminately kill all microorganisms in the process of attacking the harmful ones. This leaves the body more vulnerable to further attacks and infections.

On the following pages, *Figure 1* shows the problems associated with the bladder pain and what may have led to a weakened immune system and the effects of this on the body. *Figure 2* shows how these problems may be rectified, leading to a healthy body.

Fig. 1

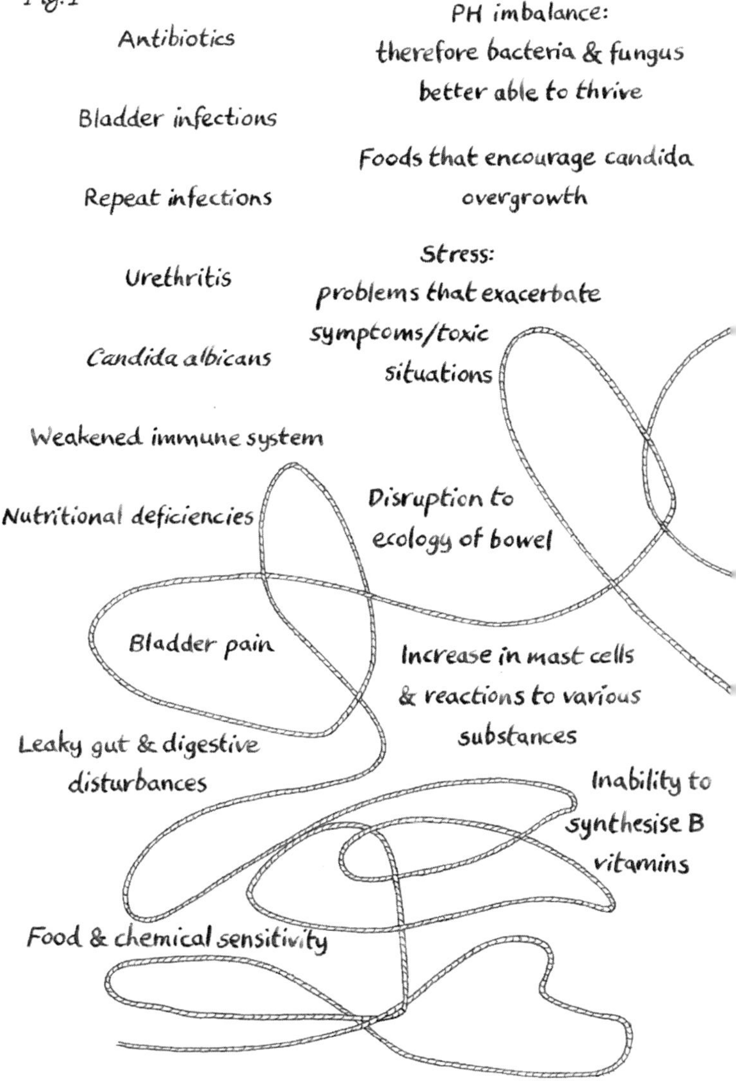

Antibiotics

PH imbalance:
therefore bacteria & fungus
better able to thrive

Bladder infections

Foods that encourage candida
overgrowth

Repeat infections

Stress:
problems that exacerbate
symptoms/toxic
situations

Urethritis

Candida albicans

Weakened immune system

Nutritional deficiencies

Disruption to
ecology of bowel

Bladder pain

Increase in mast cells
& reactions to various
substances

Leaky gut & digestive
disturbances

Inability to
synthesise B
vitamins

Food & chemical sensitivity

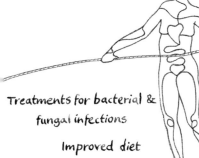

Fig.2

Kinesiology:
to determine correct
products and course of action
for body's own particular
needs

Treatments for bacterial &
fungal infections

Improved diet

Restore pH balance

Heal tissue linings

Restore ability to synthesise B
vitamins

Restore proper ability to
absorb vitamins & minerals

Probiotics:
restore ecology of bowel
and bowel function

Drinking water that is free of
contaminants

Environment:
avoidance of unnatural
chemicals that put further
strain on the immune system

Mind-body link: Input for
own personal healing, growth
& development

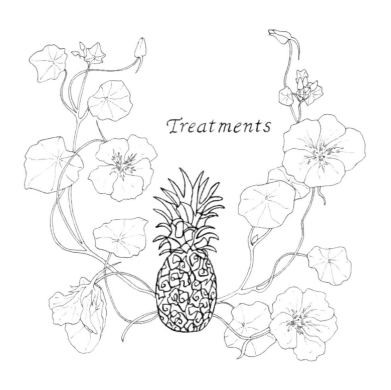

Treatments

I visited a number of alternative practitioners and received treatments including acupuncture, homeopathy, Reiki, reflexology and Chinese herbal medicine when attempting to cure the pain in my bladder. Whilst these were an extremely valuable part of the healing process, offering a holistic approach to illness and imbalances in the body (see Chapter 9), it would be hard to say which one was most helpful. Our individual circumstances are all different and we may feel more drawn to one type of treatment than another.

The two alternative forms of treatment that I am going to consider in this chapter use similar approaches and deal with what I call the 'bricks and mortar' work. They partly involve taking supplements and remedies, which are then outlined in more detail in other chapters. After all, the body has suffered injury – to the walls of the gut as well as the lining of the bladder – and this damage needs to be patched up and the main sources of the problems eliminated.

Naturopathic Treatment

One of the first alternative practitioners I saw was a naturopath. Naturopathy is a medical system that focuses on natural remedies and the body's own ability to heal and maintain itself without the use of surgery and/or drug medication.

I was asked to give a urine sample and immediately it was put under the microscope. This was connected to a TV screen on the wall above where I was sitting and the practitioner pointed out the fungi, bacteria and pieces of skin where my bladder lining had become detached. He observed that in the time it usually took for a urine test to reach a hospital laboratory much of this information would have been lost.

The naturopath explained about the problems of not only bacterial but also fungal infections, particularly the yeast and mould types of *Candida albicans* that can adapt themselves to various pH levels in the body when these are out of balance. He pointed out that many foods and drugs encourage this overgrowth, such as refined sugar, pasteurised dairy products and antibiotics. He also added that heavy metals such as amalgam fillings can cause fungus overgrowth and that once the pH levels in the body are in balance, and the heavy metal toxicity is cleared, then there is no longer an environment in which fungi and bacteria can thrive.

At the time, my symptoms had been progressing rapidly; it felt as though the process was unstoppable and the pain in my bladder was becoming worse. However, the course of naturopathic treatment that I was prescribed seemed to halt this progression. When I returned after the first course of treatment, tests showed that there were no longer bacteria or fungi present in my urine and the pH level had reduced from being very alkaline.

Looking back, I can see that most of the treatments prescribed by the naturopath correspond with treatments that I began later on, with the addition of probiotics and L-Glutamine (see Chapter 2) and an anti-candida diet (see Chapter 3).The naturopath also recommended drinking pineapple juice to help the bladder (see Chapter 6).

Kinesiology

I first visited a systematic kinesiologist five and a half years after I had developed the symptoms of interstitial cystitis. She used this method of muscle testing to identify imbalances in my body but also to check whether I would respond to certain supplements and remedies. Kinesiology comes from the Greek word *kinesis* meaning 'motion'.

Our muscles are related to the organs and systems of the body and also to the meridians or energy pathways. The practitioner asked me to resist pressure to my arm or leg as I tried to make a movement against her force. Imbalances or responses to supplements and nutrients can be detected according to whether muscles are able to resist the pressure or if they feel weak. This resistance has nothing to do with the physical strength of the muscles, and is probably something that needs to be experienced to be able to understand how it works.

Visiting a kinesiologist was a turning point in my recovery as it pinpointed what my body needed to help it get better. It meant that I was no longer taking remedies that would have little or no effect. For example, the muscle testing showed that my body would not respond to *Echinacea* but that goldenseal would be a better alternative. The practitioner also tested supplements I had bought for myself to see if they would be effective. This helped to eliminate the guesswork that tends to cause one to go around in circles. I felt I was in the hands of someone very qualified who would be able to provide a helpful treatment.

Another aspect of kinesiology is that any imbalances are treated in a certain order and testing will assess which sequence will provide the most beneficial course of treatment. The kinesiologist identified candida as one of the problems that I was suffering from and, following her dietary advice and treatment, I was surprised to find that the candida was cleared after only two or three sessions, since it had previously proved very hard to treat.

After the first session the kinesiologist prescribed Oxypro (see Chapter 3) to treat the candida, the probiotics *B. infantalis* and *L. bulgaricus*, Permatrol followed by L-Glutamine for the mucosal lining and goldenseal (see

Chapter 6) for a bacterial infection. She also observed that my liver was overloaded with a toxic metal. Over the following months I mainly continued to take L-Glutamine as well as magnesium citrate and *B. infantalis* for a shorter time. These prescriptions were determined for my body and the dosage that was appropriate for me, but it gives an idea of the course of treatment that I embarked on at this stage which proved to be extremely effective in my recovery.

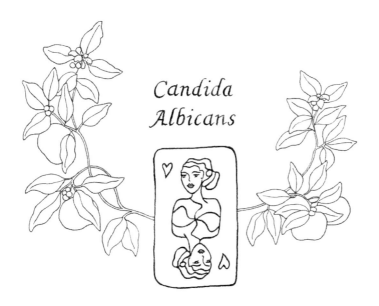

Candida Albicans

I soon became the owner of four books on *Candida Albicans* following my discovery of this parasitic yeast, which given the right conditions can proliferate inside all of us causing a variety of health problems. It must have felt very at home in my body, which was depleted of 'friendly' bacteria after my overuse of antibiotics and also given my love of sweet foods and yeasted bread. Once the ecology of the bowel has been disrupted by antibiotics the body becomes more vulnerable to candida overgrowth.

Candida is a genus of yeasts that occur naturally in the body. An overgrowth can lead to toxins that weaken the immune system, which can then produce further infections and repeated courses of antibiotics, resulting in a vicious cycle.

In his book *The Natural Way: Candida*, Simon Martin refers to Martin Crook's picture of a logical sequence of events from antibiotics to candida overgrowth which can then lead to the following effects on the body:

• Weakened immune system

• Nutritional deficiencies

• Food allergies

• Digestive disturbances involving the nervous system, endocrine system (glands) and respiratory system, and activation of viruses and parasites that had been held in check by a well nourished body....[8]

A range of symptoms can then follow such as cystitis, headaches, constipation, allergies, heartburn, anxiety and premenstrual tension. These chronic conditions are often left untreated due to the lack of recognition of candida as the source of the problem.

Candida has the ability to change from a yeast to a fungus, which is more dangerous because it develops roots, called rhizoids, which penetrate through the lining tissue of the intestinal barrier. This enables proteins from foods and toxic wastes from the infestation to begin to circulate in the bloodstream, which in turn leads to sensitivities and allergic type symptoms.

In his book on candida, Leon Chaitow suggests taking vitamin B (biotin) and restoring the bowel flora with 'potent supplements of friendly bacteria' as well as using an anti-fungal. He says that these are usually successful strategies against candida because the healthy bacteria are able to synthesise B vitamins.[9]

I wish that I had taken heed of this advice sooner as, after years of restricted diets aimed at starving the candida, as well as taking endless vitamin and mineral supplements which were most likely not being sufficiently absorbed by my leaky system, I visited a kinesiologist who put me on the correct dosage of probiotics. A vitamin B supplement was too difficult for me to take since it made the pain in my bladder much worse, but once I had started the probiotics and L-Glutamine I could then tolerate vitamin B supplements. As a result, I no longer have this problem.

Candida needs a simultaneous, multi-pronged attack: firstly, the anti-candida diet to starve the fungus; secondly, a form of anti-fungal treatment such as Citricidal or caprylic acid; thirdly, probiotics and a vitamin B supplement; finally, L-Glutamine to heal the mucous membrane of the gut.

An anti-candida programme is likely to cause a 'die-off reaction' during the time the candida is being destroyed. This can result in various reactions, such as a worsening of the original symptoms as well as headaches, upset stomach, flu-like symptoms and a white coating on the tongue. These are all signs that the anti-candida treatment is working. The advice is to start off slowly at the beginning, although there are some people who may only experience a mild die-off reaction.

For these reasons, and to help tackle the problem in the most efficient way, **it is advisable to work with a practitioner**, such as a systematic kinesiologist, naturopath, holistic medicine consultant or other health expert. Books on *Candida albicans* generally have a checklist of symptoms to help with an initial self-diagnosis followed by advice on treatment. Many books have been written on the subject but the ones I have found most useful are by Leon Chaitow and Xandria Williams, which contains a cookery guide as well as advice on various treatments (see Further Reading section).

Anti-Candida Diet

This is a strict diet aimed at starving the candida of the foods that allow it to thrive. It is therefore necessary to follow it completely in order to produce the desired effect for a period of at least three to six weeks, alongside taking probiotics and an anti-fungal.

Foods to avoid:

• Sugar: all forms of sugar including brown or white sugars, artificial sweeteners, honey, molasses, maple syrup, malt, chocolate and any form of confectionery, soft drinks including squashes, canned and fizzy drinks, icing, ice cream, desserts and puddings, cakes, biscuits and any type of food or drink that says that it contains sugar on the label.

• Fruit: raw, stewed, jams, juices, dried fruit, tinned fruit and coconut.

• Yeast: all types of breads, food with breadcrumbs, pizza base, gravy mixes, stock cubes, Bovril, Bisto, Oxo, Marmite, citric acid, and only yeast free vitamin supplements.

- Refined grains: white flour, granary flour, white rice, pasta, cornflour, custard powder and only wholegrain or wholemeal cereals.

- Fermented grains: such as soda bread and pumpernickel.

- Fermented products: beer, spirits, wine, cider, malted products, vinegar and foods containing vinegar, e.g. pickles, salad creams, soya sauce.

- Mushrooms (as they are a fungus).

- Smoked foods, such as kippers, bacon, ham, salmon, mackerel and cured meats.

- Milk and milk products.

- Hot spices and curries.

- Peanuts and peanut butter.

- Alcohol, although neat spirits may be okay.

- Dried herbs as they often contain moulds.

- Foods containing monosodium glutamate.

Oxypro

This is an additional remedy that can be used in the treatment of candida as well as for bacterial infections. Oxypro is a double-bonded oxygenating compound that has antibacterial and anti-fungal qualities and is helpful in the treatment of *Candida albicans*. When I have taken it I have felt the benefits, especially at times when my bladder has felt irritated, possibly due to a fungal infection and/or a mild bacterial infection. The product is made by Solgar and comes in a small dropper bottle. Five drops can be taken in water twice a day but it is not suitable to be taken during pregnancy.

Citricidal

Citricidal is a bitter tasting liquid concentrate made from grapefruit seed extract. It is a good anti-fungal and can be used to kill candida. It is effective against bacteria, viruses and parasites and can also be used as a mouthwash or gargle for sore throats. Higher Nature's product comes in varying bottle sizes.

Caprylic Acid

Caprylic acid is an anti-fungal derived from coconut and it is also found naturally in palm oil, butter fat and the milk of some animals, including human breast milk. It is used as a treatment for candida due to its anti-fungal properties. I was prescribed this in capsule form by the naturopath at the start of my recovery process.

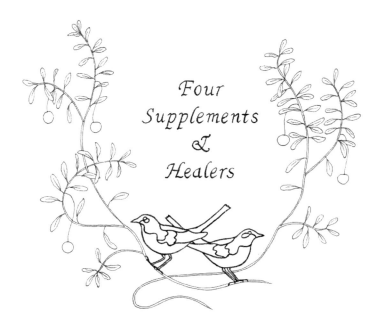

Four
Supplements
&
Healers

Magnesium

Our bodies can be deficient in magnesium due to the mineral deficient soils in which our food is often grown. We frequently hear warnings about a lack of calcium in our diets, particularly with regard to the aging process. Some foods contain the benefit of added calcium, but magnesium cannot be obtained so easily through a healthy diet. The two are required by the body to work together since the body's muscles need calcium to contract and magnesium to relax, and they need to be in balance for the cells to function properly.

A magnesium deficiency can be indicated in any spastic condition (muscles going in spasm) such as cystitis, asthma, migraine, colitis, angina, chronic back pain, hypertension, tremors and seizures. In addition, symptoms such as feeling dizzy, confused, depressed, irritable or abnormally aggressive can also be attributed to a magnesium deficiency since the breakdown of brain chemicals and hormones is dependent on this mineral. Stress can also reduce the levels of magnesium in the body.

One of the symptoms of interstitial cystitis is an increase in mast cells inside the bladder. These cells play an important role in any type of allergic response, each one releasing mediator chemicals when an allergen is present and thereby bringing about an allergic response. An example of this is sneezing as a result of hay fever, but generally an allergic response will involve inflammation in the affected part of the body. A magnesium deficiency causes the mast cells to release more histamine, so correcting this can also do its part in improving the symptoms of bladder pain.

The kinesiologist I saw told me that I was very deficient in magnesium. I then took it in a powder form known as magnesium citrate, and I continue to take it every so often. I believe that taking magnesium played a major part in my recovery and has also helped to improve my overall health.

Probiotics

Probiotics will be to the medicine in the twenty-first century as antibiotics and microbiology were in the twentieth.[10]

Alexander Fleming discovered penicillin in the late 1920s and by the 1950s penicillin antibiotics were being used to cure all kinds of deadly diseases. However, these drugs are generally becoming less effective since many bacteria have developed resistance to them.

We are now hearing much more about probiotics and adverts have appeared on our television screens for probiotic products such as drinks and yoghurts, although many of these products contain only a very small proportion of the necessary bacteria.

Antibiotics are used to kill microorganisms, especially bacteria, but are indiscriminate in the ones that they kill. Probiotics are made up of live, friendly bacteria that can maintain or restore health. Even when one is not taking antibiotics they can be hard to fully avoid since the animals we eat are often routinely fed antibiotics. These are used as a way not only to control disease but also to increase the growing rate of animals.

The three main types of friendly bacteria are *Lactobacillus acidophilus*, *Bifidobacterium bifidum* and *Lactobacillus bulgaricus*. Sufficient numbers of these bacteria are required in our bodies to prevent a wide range of health problems – including providing protection against urinary tract infections. They are also effective in treating candida overgrowth and can help in eliminating the effects of toxins and environmental pollutants that we encounter in our daily lives.

Natasha Trenev has done much high-tech research into the health benefits of probiotic cultures and has written a book called *Probiotics: Nature's Internal Healers*. Her advice is: 'To bring candida back to manageable levels, nothing is more important than probiotics.[11]

I took probiotics, mainly *B. infantalis* and *L. bulgaricus*, which are found naturally in the gastrointestinal tract of human infants and inhibit the effects of some strains of *E. coli* bacteria as well as producing important B complex vitamins and helping with the absorption of calcium and other vitamins and minerals. *L. bulgaricus* is a transient bacterium but it helps with the colonisation of resident healthy bacteria in the intestines and it is a good detoxifier.

I continue to take the probiotic *Lactobacillus acidophilus*, by BioCare. They also make a probiotic powder called Concentrated Cranberry, which can be an effective treatment for a cystitis infection and is made up of cranberry concentrate together with *L. acidophilus*. Cranberries contain a compound that stops harmful bacteria from attaching themselves to the tissues of the bladder lining. Cranberry juice has a naturally bitter taste so commercial varieties usually contain added sugar which would counteract the benefits and therefore is not helpful in the case of an infection.

I also recently discovered a probiotic range by Dr Udo Erasmus. I take Super 5 Oral Health, which is a blend of five probiotics in raspberry flavoured lozenges. Another good probiotic is Trenev Trio, which contains the three main types of bacteria in one capsule. These are quite expensive but could be taken as a one-off to boost the immune system. They can be obtained from Revital Health in London.

If you need to take antibiotics it is recommended that you take probiotics for two weeks following completion of the course.

L-Glutamine

L-Glutamine is an amino acid that is important for gut barrier function and health and which can promote healing and encourage the absorptive capacity of the intestines. Levels of glutamine can become depleted through stress and without it immune cells cannot function correctly. In his book *The Natural Way: Candida*, Simon Martin highly recommends taking this amino acid as a supplement since it is the main nutrient needed to repair fast growing cells in the intestinal tract, helping to heal the damage that candida has caused in the gut. It can reduce inflammation, correct nutritional deficiencies and digestive efficiency.[12]

Candida albicans, in its fungal form, can cause damage to organ walls causing them to become 'leaky'. When damage is caused to the intestinal lining it can lead to an increased permeability known as 'leaky gut syndrome'. For this Leon Chaitow prescribes L-Glutamine as well as recommending Permatrol made by BioCare.[13] Permatrol contains L-Glutamine and N-Acetylglucosamine (NAG) which aids in the formation of connective tissues lining the intestinal tract and helps to protect the underlying tissues.

I took this as a supplement in capsule form over a period of two years, after visiting the kinesiologist who prescribed it for me in the correct dose. I then took it again for a short while a year later and I still buy it occasionally to take as a top-up.

Urine Therapy

Urine has been used as a healing agent in practically all civilisations and cultures. It seemingly dies only to reappear again time after time.[14]

This aspect of my treatment is hard to write about but it made such a dramatic difference to my health that I feel compelled to do so. One day, during my illness, I walked into a health food shop and a yellow booklet on the shelf caught my eye. It was called *Urine-Therapy: It May Save Your Life* by Dr Beatrice Bartnett. The booklet describes urine therapy as a 'very ancient and drugless form of intrinsic medicine',[15] and states that any disease, except those caused by trauma or structural defects, can be healed using this form of treatment.

Prior to finding out about urine therapy, I had received some treatment called BICOM® Resonance Therapy. The practitioner I saw had described a very complicated method of devising a homeopathic remedy using urine from a patient suffering from similar bladder problems to myself.

However, urine therapy turns out to be the simplest form of homeopathy that exists: it involves taking a small amount of your own urine or, as my kinesiologist prescribed for me, 1–5 drops under the tongue for the first day, 5–10 drops in the morning on the second day, and then 5–10 drops morning and evening for four weeks thereafter.

This may sound repugnant but urine is a sterile fluid which has been removed from the blood by the kidneys and the toxins have already been removed by the liver. It consists of 95% water and 5% other substances including vitamins, minerals, proteins, enzymes, hormones, antibodies and amino acids.

There is **a strong caution given against using urine therapy with prescription drugs, over-the-counter or recreational drugs**.

When I first tried urine therapy I had what is called a 'healing crisis', which can happen with any natural healing therapy. For me this was a brief and sudden stomach upset but each person may react, if at all, in different ways. The 'healing crisis' occurs because of the detoxification process in the body during which any stored toxins or pre-existing diseases, which Dr Bartnett says may go back to an early childhood disease, will be released.[16] The toxins may be eliminated through the skin or the bowel, flu-like symptoms may occur as well as headaches, rashes, nausea or diarrhoea.

Although my health had already improved somewhat, I was still suffering from a chronic bladder condition at the time I tried urine therapy and the improvements that then followed were very clear to me. I was willing to try anything to aid my recovery but I know that others may be more wary.

Some of the individuals written about in Dr Bartnett's case studies also mention a book called *The Water of Life* by J. W. Armstrong, which was first published in the 1950s but a new edition was printed in 2005.

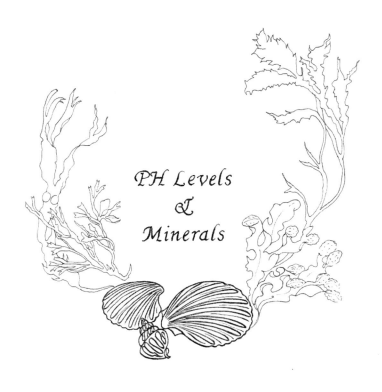

PH Levels & Minerals

The pH scale runs from 0 to 14 with pure water at the midpoint of 7 and anything below 7 being acid and above 7 alkaline. The ideal pH level for our body is a slightly alkaline 7.3, so maintaining a balance between acidity and alkalinity is important for our health. If the body's fluids are too acid then alkaline minerals will be sought to readdress the balance, and if too little of these are available from our diets, they will be taken directly from the body, such as the liver, muscles, bones and so on.

Our bodies produce acid waste as a by-product of normal cell activity and this can be excreted harmlessly in the form of carbon dioxide and water, unless there is an excess of acid which forms a residue called 'acid ash'. Minerals are alkaline substances used to buffer this acid residue. These minerals are now in reduced supply in the soil due to intensive farming methods over recent decades. Organic fruit and vegetables may be equally deficient in minerals as non-organic foods for this reason.

As described in Chapter 2, the naturopath I saw described how we are more susceptible to fungal and bacterial infections if the pH of the body is out of balance. Minerals are alkaline forming and help our bodies in many ways, such as cell growth and healing as well as assisting in the elimination of toxins.

Higher Nature sell a product called UltraTrace which is a trace mineral supplement taken from the Great Salt Lake in Utah which contains minute amounts of seventy-nine naturally occurring minerals in a form that can be easily absorbed by the body. Sea vegetables (see Chapter 10) and blue-green algae are also very rich in minerals.

Klamlath Lake Blue Green Algae

Algae are a form of phytoplankton which grow naturally in oceans or fresh water and contain an abundance of minerals and vitamins that can be easily absorbed by the body, since their cell walls are soft and easy to digest. They can help to support the immune system, correct the pH balance of the body when it is too acidic and prevent or reverse anaemia. They are also very high in protein and can therefore be a good alternative to eating meat and dairy products. When I have taken blue-green algae I find that my desire to eat sweet foods diminishes.

Klamlath Lake is situated 3,000 feet up in the Cascade Mountains of Oregon in the United States. The algae found growing there are as a result of volcanic eruptions which deposited millions of tons of mineral-rich volcanic ash across the land.

The suggested dosage for algae is to start with a small amount, about a quarter of a teaspoon, before building up slowly to a daily maximum of 2 teaspoons. The blue-green algae can be bought as either a powder, which can be mixed with water or juice and made into a drink, or else it can be taken in capsule form. I usually buy the 30g container of the powder and take about a half a teaspoon per day.

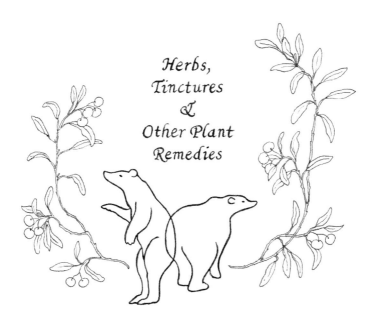

Herbs,
Tinctures
&
Other Plant
Remedies

Herbs and Tinctures

Herbal remedies have been used in all cultures for many thousands of years. Their medicinal properties help to combat disease but also support the body's own natural healing processes.

The following is a list of herbal remedies that I have found useful in helping to heal my bladder, as well as those that I continue to use at those times when I feel the symptoms of a urinary tract infection or else as a preventative against further infections. Herbs such as marshmallow, chamomile and nettle can be used as part of the healing process for a damaged and sensitive bladder whereas others, such as buchu, juniper and uva-ursi have anti-microbial properties for killing bacteria in the case of an infection.

Infusions can be made with fresh leaves steeped in hot water for 5–10 minutes and then strained and drunk 3–6 times a day. A general guide for quantities is to use two teaspoons of a dried herb to a cupful of water or one tablespoon to a pint of water. The quantity can be doubled if using fresh herbs.

Decoctions are made with the roots of herbs where about 25 g (1 oz) can be simmered in a pint of water for ten minutes and then strained and drunk.

The effects of herbs can be powerful and care needs to be taken. However, most herbs can generally be used for a period of three to six weeks followed by a break of a couple of weeks before resuming, if necessary. More information on herbal remedies can be obtained from the National Institute of Medical Herbalists, including a list of herbal practitioners.

Bearberry/Uva-Ursi

Uva-ursi is a plant that thrives on the rocky mountainous slopes of the northern hemisphere and its name means 'bear's grapes' since bears probably ate the small red fruits. It was considered one of the best remedies for urinary tract infections until the 1940s when it was overtaken by antibiotics.

The fresh herb Uva-ursi Complex tincture by A.Vogel can be taken for the symptoms of a bladder infection. Alfred Vogel's remedies are made by Bioforce.

I have also used Uva Ursi and Juniper Formula by Solgar, containing a combination of extracts of uva-ursi leaf, juniper berry, buchu leaf, parsley herb and barberry fruit, which comes in vegetable capsules. Avoiding acidic foods including fruit and juices helps the herbs to work but bearberry/uva-ursi should be taken for no longer than a period of one week.

Another good remedy containing uva-ursi is made by Arkopharma but it is not available to buy in shops in the UK. It can be bought over the internet from ParaSend (www.parasend.com) and comes as a liquid in little glass phials which also contain a combination of nettle, heather and birch extracts. The French version of this Arkopharma remedy is called Phytofluide Urinair Comfort and the Italian version is called Arkofluidi Sinergia Depura.

Buchu

Buchu is a shrub that is native to South Africa and grows wild in the mountains. It was traditionally used by indigenous people as a stimulating tonic and diuretic but it has a long history as a remedy for urinary tract infections. In the late eighteenth century it was prescribed for cystitis, nephritis and urethritis (inflammation of bladder, kidneys and urethra). The leaves are strongly aromatic and contain a volatile oil which gives it an aniseed flavour. Unlike most teas, the small leaves are steeped in cold water (rather than hot) before drinking.

Chamomile

Chamomile is a plant that comes from the daisy family and is native to Europe and parts of Asia. The flowers can be used to make soothing teas for any irritating conditions since chamomile contains active constituents with anti-inflammatory properties. Chamomile tea can also be taken to help promote sleep.

Goldenseal

Goldenseal is a herb belonging to the buttercup family and was traditionally used by Native American Indians to treat digestive problems, inflammation, liver disorders, fever and loss of appetite. It is a healer for inflamed mucus membranes and can also be used as a remedy for a number of problems including candida, catarrhal infections and other infections due to its antibiotic and anti-fungal nature. For this reason it is advisable to supplement with probiotics if using goldenseal for any length of time. The advice is to use this herb with caution and not during pregnancy.

Juniper

Juniper is a hardy evergreen conifer with needle-like leaves and small berries that are used in the making of gin. Juniper berries have long been used for their medicinal properties, particularly as a diuretic and antiseptic, but they also contain substances known to combat bacteria and viruses. Juniper must be avoided in pregnancy or if suffering from kidney disease.

Whilst suffering an *Enterococcus* bladder infection that was hard to treat, I resorted to taking two types of antibiotics.

My great aunt had apparently sworn by drinking gin as a way of combating a cystitis infection but in the past I had never found this to be helpful. However, in the case of the *Enterococcus* infection I found that gin reduced the irritating symptoms. When I did some research on the internet I found that juniper is thought to be effective against *Enterococcus* bacteria in particular.

Marshmallow

In the UK marshmallow is usually associated with soft pink or white sweets but it is also the name of a wild plant with pale pink flowers that is native to Europe and western Asia and grows in marshy, wet places. Preparations from the roots, leaves and stems have traditionally been used to soothe inflammation both inside and outside the body. The plant contains a high concentration of mucilage in the root and it can soothe irritated membranes in the urinary tract as well as the gut and lungs. It was infusions made from marshmallow root that I used the most in my recovery to help heal my bladder.

Nettle

The stinging nettle, one of the most common British native plants, is easy to find and is a sign of soil fertility. Nettles can help to ease inflammation of the urinary tract since they contain polysaccharides (energy-rich carbohydrates produced by a combination of sugar molecules). Nettles can be used to make tea infusions or they can be used in cooking, such as nettle soup. It is best to pick young, fresh leaves from the tops of the plants.

Oregano

Oregano is a herb that is native to the Mediterranean and southern and central Asia where it has been used as a traditional medicine for thousands of years due to its anti-microbial properties. Its Latin name *Origanum vulgare* derives from the Greek meaning 'joy of the mountains'. Wild oregano oil can be used to treat all kinds of infection as it is antibacterial, anti-parasitic, anti-fungal and anti-viral and, when consumed, it can get to any area of the body.

Sweet Cures produce a Wild Oregano Oil C80 that is made from wild oregano and retains the full effect of its chemical components. Four to eight drops can be taken with a small of amount milk (or an alternative to milk) and a little honey, but I found this to be a strong oil and **it may be advisable to exercise caution when using it**. Another way I have tried using the oil is to have a sitz bath, where a few drops are added to a bowl of water which can then be sat in, again using caution with the number of drops due to the oil's strength.

Chinese Herbal Medicine

Chinese herbal medicine has been used to treat different types of illnesses over many centuries in China and the East. It is based on the concept of yin and yang and therefore aims to treat according to signs and symptoms that reflect an imbalance in the body.

I was recommended a Chinese herbalist who uses the traditional method of prescribing a mixture of dried herbs to boil up into a drink, which I took over the course of a couple of weeks before returning for a second appointment. At the start I was asked to give an account of my medical history and any health problems and symptoms that I was suffering from. There are about three hundred herbs to choose from, so I did not know which ones I was using but I felt that this treatment helped with the pain in my bladder as well as my overall health at that time.

The taste of Chinese herbs is known to be unusual and bitter so they take a little getting used to in the beginning. The herbs can also be taken in the form of pills or tinctures which is the modern method of treatment.

Other plant remedies

Aloe vera

Aloe vera is a tropical, succulent plant that has been used for thousands of years for its health-giving properties. It has long pointed leaves containing fleshy tissue for storing water so that it can withstand periods of drought. It is this fleshy tissue from within the leaves that has beneficial properties for health, as it contains essential minerals, vitamins, proteins, amino acids, lipids, enzymes and polysaccharides. Amongst other benefits, including helping with detoxification of the tissues and maintaining a healthy colon, *Aloe vera* is reputed to heal both internal and external wounds due to mucinous polysaccharides, which are important for the health of lining tissues in the body. It also has an alkalinising effect on the body.

Forever Living sell an *Aloe vera* drink and have independent distributors up and down the UK, but it is also possible to make a fresh *Aloe vera* juice from the live plant. I do this by slicing the length of the leaf and scooping out the tissue from inside with a metal spoon and then putting this in a liquidiser with a cup of water. I keep this in the fridge and use it as a concentrate to make into a drink to take over a few days.

Pineapple

When I visited a naturopath in the early stages of my bladder illness, he advised me to drink pineapple juice. The most active compound in pineapple is bromelain, which was discovered in 1876 and found to have anti-inflammatory effect by inhibiting or blocking substances that increase swelling and pain. It can also help to speed up the healing of damaged tissues. When I went out for a drink I would often ask for a pineapple juice, or pineapple and soda, instead of having alcohol or anything else that I knew might trigger pain in my bladder.

D-Mannose

D-Mannose is a natural treatment for bladder infections and offers an alternative to taking antibiotics. Mannose is a natural sugar found in the body as well as in wood and in minute quantities in some fruits and *Aloe vera*. It works as a treatment for bladder infections by attracting the bacteria that would otherwise adhere to the bladder wall, which are then flushed out of the system along with the urine. People with a healthy bladder will usually have enough mannose naturally in their urine, whilst others may not.

D-Mannose can be bought either in a white powder or tablet form, called Waterfall D-Mannose, from Sweet Cures. This is a family business which sells mannose extracted from sweet forest timbers without using solvents and can guarantee a 100% natural product.

When I was suffering from an *Enterococcus* infection that was proving very hard to treat, I contacted Sweet Cures via email and they gave me some very helpful and knowledgeable advice. They also sell Xylotene which is another natural sugar that is useful against *Streptococcus* infections and can be used in conjunction with D-Mannose for infections where there may be more than one bacterium present. Xylotene also helps to maintain healthy teeth, gums, joints and bones.

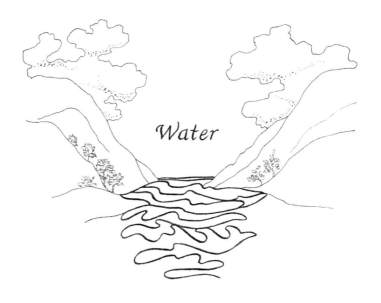

The body is very much like a sponge and is composed of trillions of chambers called cells that hold liquid. The quality of our life is directly connected to the quality of our water.[17]

Water is an important element of our lives and perhaps one that we take for granted with such a ready supply in the UK. Water quality can vary dramatically from one source to another but without it we would not be alive, since it makes up to 75% of our body weight and is needed to hydrate and cleanse our cells and tissues.

Drinking water in Britain went through a period of revolution after a clear link between sewage leeching into London's Broad Street well and cholera outbreaks in the city had been identified by John Snow in 1854. From the

1950s onwards there have been new problems such as oxygen depletion, acidification and contamination from heavy metals, nitrates, bacteria and toxic substances, including chlorine, lead and xenoestrogens. Xenoestrogens are chemicals that provoke or mimic oestrogen in the body, and occur in many pesticides and insecticides, chemicals found in plastics and some food preservatives. Much of the problem has been due to agricultural methods where pesticides and chemical fertilisers have run off farmland into rivers and also entered the groundwater. Water purification methods are not wholly effective and some pollutants in our drinking water may go undetected.

Dr Masaru Emoto has done studies on the diversity of the molecular structure of water and how this is not only affected by contaminants such as pollution and toxic wastes, but also by energy and vibrations in the environment; if these are positive they can help water to become energised and return to its original life-giving state. He looks at the crystalline structures of frozen water, which form patterns like those we think of as a traditional snowflake pattern, but with polluted water these structures will show distorted or randomly formed crystalline shapes.[18]

Early on in my illness I bought myself a water distiller since I found that drinking water from any other source, including bottled water, caused varying degrees of irritation to my bladder. Steam distillation is a way to produce pure water that is free of contaminants such as chemicals, pollutants and chlorine. Water is heated and turned to steam which rises and leaves behind any contaminants. The steam is then condensed back into pure water for drinking.

I pour my water into a ceramic jug through a funnel containing a metal spiral or vortex to energise the water. I then use a technique suggested by Dr Emoto (who has written several books on the topic) of sending positive energy to improve the molecular structure of the water. I think this does make a difference.

Water distillers can be bought from Greens Water Systems and they also offer a range of other products to help produce healthy drinking water. This is a cheaper and more environmentally sustainable method than buying bottled water.

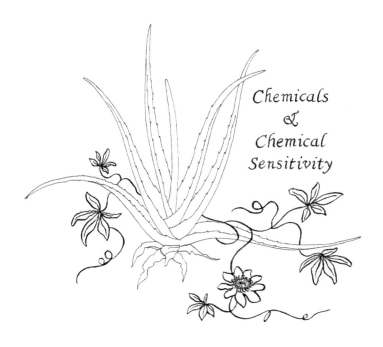

Chemicals
&
Chemical
Sensitivity

Chronic poisoning occurs when repeated small doses of a toxic substance are absorbed over a long period. It is often difficult to detect and its symptoms may be ascribed to completely different causes.[19]

In 1951 Dr Theron Randolph discovered chemical sensitivity. All living things are made up of chemicals but it is the manmade or synthetic varieties that are harmful to our health since the enzymes in our bodies designed to deal with naturally occurring chemicals often struggle with these additional foreign invaders.

I first became aware that I was chemically sensitive when I used an antibacterial soap containing synthetic chemicals. Each time I used the soap I noticed that I felt nauseous almost instantaneously, but I simply stopped using the soap rather than understanding that this may have been a signal of something more serious. These liquid soaps are now extremely popular and I still try to avoid them.

It was shortly after this that I developed the symptoms of interstitial cystitis. I was also regularly doing silk painting using chemical dyes at this time. I had noticed that my urethritis seemed to become worse and I needed to empty my bladder more frequently when I had been working in the studio where I was painting. I now understand that I was reacting to the chemicals that I was using and because of my work I could identify a clear link. However, we are all being exposed to an unprecedented number of chemicals in our environment and in our food. It is the combination of these chemicals that makes them all the more harmful:

Chemicals can combine in the environment to form other substances, which may be more or less toxic than the original materials. Once absorbed by living organisms, two or more compounds can exert combined effects much greater than the sum of their individual toxicities.[20]

Nine months after I had developed the burning pain in my bladder, I bought a book called *Tired or Toxic?* by Sherry Rogers. In this book she writes about detoxification pathways and the bottlenecks created in the body by an overload of toxins. Rogers makes the link between candida problems and chemical sensitivity, since to be metabolised candida needs to pass through the same pathways in the body as other triggers such as pesticides, sugar and exhaust fumes as well as other chemicals, such as pollutants, additives, paints, varnishes, air fresheners, perfumes, tobacco smoke and disinfectants, to name but a few. [21] Therefore, by treating candida the toxic overload is reduced and we can become dramatically less food or chemically sensitive. This is certainly something that I experienced, and the pain triggered in my bladder gradually decreased after the candida was treated.

The brain is the primary target organ for chemicals causing symptoms of foggy headedness, tiredness, lethargy, confusion and so on. On top of this, the body makes many brain chemicals (neurotransmitters) that control mood and memory which also need to be metabolised. Other affected organs vary from person to person, which is probably why there is no obvious link made between the symptoms, such as a burning in the bladder in my case, and chemical sensitivity. The signs are not constant or often even properly noticed until we have reached overload.

Metabolism is highly individual and for some people it is very hard to get rid of harmful compounds. A deficiency in the enzymes that the body uses to deal with toxic chemicals may be the root of the problem for some, which makes us more vulnerable to their effects. But we are all at risk of damage caused by chemicals that are known to trigger problems such as irritation, disruption to the endocrine system, mood changes and are potentially carcinogenic.

N-acetylcysteine

N-acetylcysteine (NAC) is an amino acid produced by the body which helps to synthesise a powerful antioxidant called glutathione. As a result, NAC can be used to remove heavy metal toxins, such as lead and mercury, from the body. NAC binds to the toxic heavy metals before removing them, so it protects against illness as well as helping to restore health following free radical damage.

When taking NAC it is necessary also to take a supplement of trace minerals, including zinc, since it increases the excretion of zinc and other minerals from the body. In addition, it is recommended to take three times the amount of vitamin C supplement to the amount of NAC being taken.

I noticed a marked improvement in my health and energy levels, following pesticide poisoning, when I took a supplement of NAC.

Dental Amalgam/Mercury

It is rarely possible to define a lethal dose of a poison. Since all individuals in a natural population of animals (or plants for that matter) differ slightly from each other, the effect of a given dose of poison will vary from one individual to another.[22]

A little while ago I heard a radio programme on mercury, which talked about the origin of the term 'mad as a hatter'. In the eighteenth century hat makers used mercury in the making of hats to soften the fur fibres for the felt. In the process they breathed in the mercury vapours causing them to become poisoned and go mad.

Mercury is a cumulative poison but nevertheless there has been much doubt and debate on the potentially harmful effects of using amalgam, which contains a mixture of mercury, in fillings.

In 1999 I went for a test with a dental practitioner who was the President of the British Society for Mercury Free Dentistry, to discover whether or not I was sensitive to mercury. Dr. Jack Levenson wrote a book on this subject called *Menace in the Mouth* which was published in 2000. When I visited his dental practice I was given information in a handout stating that research clearly demonstrates that mercury vapour is released from amalgam fillings and that 'this point is no longer a matter of dispute'. A 1997 publication by the British Dental Association states that 'about 3% of the population are estimated to suffer from mercury sensitivity'.[23]

The tests showed that I was sensitive to mercury and I had quite number of amalgam fillings in my teeth at the time. I had these removed by my own dentist using a plan set up by the practitioner who took the sensitivity test. This gave guidance on how to protect the patient from mercury vapour during treatment and also the sequence in which the fillings should be removed. I can't say that I noticed a marked improvement following the removal of my mercury fillings but I feel satisfied that I have eliminated a major toxic element from my body, which I am sure has contributed to my recovery.

In her book *Along the Healing Path: Recovering from Interstitial Cystitis*, Catherine Simone writes about the toxicity factor of mercury fillings and the process of removing these toxins effectively. She explains that it takes time for the poison to clear out of the system and used colostrums to cleanse the mercury from her body. She expressed an immediate feeling of improvement.[24] Colostrum is the milk produced by mammals to feed to their offspring for the first few hours after giving birth and it is especially high in nutrients and antibodies. Supplements of colostrum can be bought and these are usually made from bovine colostrum. I have recently taken this and have felt the benefits of this supplement.

Toothpaste

Powders for cleaning teeth were used by the Egyptians up to 4,000 thousand years ago and others made from various substances, including crushed bones, chalk and shells, had been used by civilisations for hundreds of years before glycerine was first used to make a paste early in the nineteenth century. Toothpaste began to be mass produced in 1873 and became more popular after the Second World War.

In recent decades synthetic agents have been added to toothpaste including sodium lauryl sulphate, which is a powerful and toxic chemical detergent, and triclosan, for its anti-bacterial properties. Fluoride can be harmful too, in some cases causing dental fluorosis where the visible sign of overexposure to fluoride is shown in the teeth, but there is also concern around the effects of daily doses of this substance on other body tissues.

For several years I have used Green People's toothpaste made with natural ingredients such as fennel and propolis. Propolis is a substance gathered by bees to keep their hives sterile. The toothpaste therefore has antibacterial properties and can help with gum problems.

It is free from fluoride and synthetic additives and I have not needed to have any new fillings in my teeth since I began using it.

Chemicals in Food

Overuse, misuse and abuse of pesticides has caused human ill health and suffering, and has exhausted soils and increased insect resistance to pesticides.[25]

Chemicals in the form of pesticides and additives are consumed daily in our food – many people are thought to ingest at least a hundred different synthetic chemicals each day. Information from the Pesticide Action Network UK says that, on average, 30% of the food purchased by the British public contains pesticide residues.[26]

The pain in my bladder used to become worse when I had eaten food containing additives and preservatives, but it would have been impossible for me to identify which ones exactly were triggering the pain. I avoided foods containing additives or preservatives for a long time and continue to eat organic food as much as possible, although I no longer have a noticeable reaction to the foods containing additives.

The body contains an array of enzymes that deal with naturally occurring chemicals, including those in natural foods that we eat and which would otherwise be harmful and toxic without this detoxification system in place. These enzymes have evolved over time and been inherited through our ancestors since they are passed on from parent to child. The enzymes that deal with these natural chemicals can also work on synthetic or manufactured chemicals, so long as they are not overwhelmed by the quantity.[27]

Of course, it is impossible to tell quite how tainted foods are with these substances and the effects they may have on our bodies. Pesticides need extra metabolic energy from the body to be processed, therefore overworking the detox system and causing a further depletion of vital nutrients that the body needs in order to be able to function efficiently.

Children are more vulnerable to the toxic effects of organophosphate pesticides because they have significantly lower levels of an enzyme called paraoxonase to protect them until at least the age of seven.[28] Some individuals are more susceptible to pesticides and other chemicals due to an enzyme deficiency, which explains why certain people are more chemically sensitive than others.[29]

The term 'pesticide' covers a wide range of substances used against living organisms which compete for our food or carry disease. The main categories are insecticides, herbicides and fungicides. As more of these chemicals have been utilised, resistance to them has developed, leading to the necessity of using even more powerful chemicals. Organic farming does not use synthetic pesticides and employs methods that improve soil fertility.

The Pesticide Action Network UK website (www.pan-uk.org) offers a downloadable booklet, called *Pesticides on a Plate*, giving information on pesticides and a guide on how to avoid them. Organic food tends to be more expensive and, in acknowledgement of this, advice is given to start buying organic produce for the foods that you eat most often or those that may be more likely to contain chemical residues. The website has a section on assessments of residues in foods and these are updated to give consumers an idea of which foods currently contain the most pesticides.

Advice is also given on growing your own food. About four years after I had developed a painful bladder I took on an allotment where now I grow my own fruit and vegetables, which I know are safe from pesticides and any other chemicals. It is hard work and can be frustrating at times when crops do not grow or the potatoes and tomatoes get blight, but the benefits far outweigh any of the difficulties. These rewards are as much to do with spending time close to nature and providing nourishment for the soul as about producing organic food, not to mention the reduction in food miles.

Chemicals in Food Packaging

A few years ago I watched a television programme about scientists who were carrying out research into why alligators in Florida's Everglades were experiencing difficulty in reproducing – they were laying eggs that failed to hatch and, in some cases, were producing hermaphrodite young. You may wonder what a story about alligators has to do with how we package our food, but the scientists discovered that the fertility problems were being caused by chemicals found in the water that are especially used in packaging materials, including plastic water bottles.

A while later I was working in a school and read in a textbook about hormone disruption in humans caused by certain chemicals; it turns out that it has been known for a long time that compounds such as bisphenol A, which are widely used in the making of bottles and containers, disrupt the human sex hormones, but can also be very harmful to our health in other ways. These chemicals, often referred to as 'gender benders', are endocrine-disrupting chemicals. The endocrine system includes not only sex hormones but is made up of a collection of glands that produce hormones in the pituitary and thyroid glands. Disruption in these areas leads to a whole host of other health problems. The chemicals not only affect humans but also other living organisms in the environment.

Food from supermarkets is often over-packaged to give the impression that it might somehow be more healthy, fresh and less contaminated by anything around it, but chemicals in the packaging itself can be harmful. At home food can be stored in the fridge in a ceramic bowl or dish with a plate on top or put into a glass jar, since these containers are made of inert substances. In other words they hold on to their molecules. Parchment or greaseproof paper can be used as an alternative to cling film.

For many years I have used a stainless steel 'tiffin' box to carry my lunch to work (see chapter 10). In Britain today lunch for workers is typically food that has been packaged or wrapped in a plastic container and bought from a shop. Foods can pick up the plastic molecules, particularly those that are heated in a plastic container, especially with foods that are more acidic.

Chemical Air Pollution

[P]ollution seeps under barbed wire and falls from the sky beyond the limits of the highest brick walls. It flows down rivers and it can be found in the deepest recesses of the oceans or in the snows of the uninhabited Arctic wastes.[30]

For many centuries humans have had to deal with different forms of environmental pollution, with some of the biggest changes taking place during the industrial revolution. Until the middle of the nineteenth century the main sources of pollution were from the domestic burning of fuel and the production of iron, steel and chemicals. Nowadays it is the effect and scale of our consumer society and patterns of consumption that are a major cause of pollution. An overload of pollutants in the environment has a direct toxic effect on all living creatures, including ourselves.

The Environment Act 1995 required the UK government to produce a national air quality strategy containing standards and objectives for the first time. These were derived from EU Air Quality Directives which identified twelve pollutants including sulphur dioxide, nitrogen dioxide, carbon monoxide, benzene, nickel and mercury.[31]

As mentioned above, the pain in my bladder became worse when I breathed in the chemical fumes from the silk paints that I was working with, and due to my chemical sensitivity I was also affected by chemicals in cigarette smoke, air fresheners, paints and all types of sprays, including perfume. It is possible to reduce our exposure to these kinds of contaminants by trying to avoid them in the home, but the bigger picture of environmental air pollution is more difficult to escape from. The lungs are a sensitive organ and can be damaged by pollution as well as by high levels of stress.

We may think that we have little influence over the levels of airborne toxins that we may be exposed to in our daily lives, but a man called Dr Bill Wolverton conducted studies for NASA on plants as an effective way of removing toxins as well as balancing humidity levels in the home. Plants can absorb potentially harmful pollutants such as formaldehyde, benzene, ammonia and carbon monoxide. Dr Wolverton has written a book, published by Penguin in 1997, called *How to Grow Fresh Air: 50 Houseplants that Purify Your Home or Office*.

I have a number of plants in my home but the two that are well known to have a beneficial effect are the Peace Lily and the Madagascar Dragon Tree (*Draecaena marginata*). Other effective air cleansing house plants are the Boston Fern, Bamboo Palm, Chinese Evergreen, English Ivy, Gerbera Daisy and Dwarf Date Palm.

Chemicals in Household Products

Many household cleaners are a source of chemicals that may cause harm due to contact with the skin or through inhalation, particularly air fresheners and furniture sprays, but also cleaning materials such as white spirit, turpentine, methylated spirit, polish, bleach, aerosols and oven cleaners. Paints and varnishes give off strong chemicals, as do vinyl flooring and some carpets and furnishings, although these may not be such an obvious source of problems.

Natural products for cleaning, including the Ecover range, can be found online or through some supermarket chains and health food shops. An alternative and safe method is to use vinegar which has been known for many years to be an efficient cleaning fluid.

Chemicals in Toiletries and Cosmetic Products

The skin is seen as the third lung and breathes just as surely and necessarily as the lungs themselves.[32]

The skin is the largest organ of the body and provides the outermost covering for our internal organs and protection against such things as unwanted bacteria and harmful rays of sunlight. The thickness varies for different parts of the body with some areas, like the soles of our feet, being thicker than others. Men have thicker skin than women. The outer layer of the skin (the epidermis) contains cells to produce keratin, the same hard protein substance that our nails are made from, and a fatty substance to make the skin waterproof. The layer beneath (the dermis) contains the hair follicles, glands, blood vessels, lymph vessels and nerves.

Some 60% of what we put on our skin will be absorbed into the blood stream. In recent years rising numbers of new synthetic chemicals have been developed and added to toiletries and cosmetic products. Parabens are still legal in the UK and are commonly used as preservatives in cosmetic products. Parabens occur naturally in nature but they are also produced synthetically for commercial use and a big area of concern is their possible link to breast cancer.

Although it may not be possible to avoid all of these chemicals, contact with them can be minimised by using products that are organic or contain as many natural ingredients as possible. Neal's Yard Remedies, Dr Hauschka, Avalon Organics and JASON all provide a range of skincare and other products that use organic ingredients that are not tested on animals. Bio-Life have created an advanced natural skincare range called MediCleanse for those who suffer from allergies. The Healthy House also provide a range of unscented products for allergy sufferers.

In Traditional Chinese Medicine the lungs and large intestine are partner organs, both being responsible for eliminating waste products from our bodies. The skin is also connected with these organs. If the large intestine is not functioning effectively then toxins will begin to be discharged through the skin, which also helps to rid the body of wastes.

A healthy diet and well functioning internal organs, particularly the large intestine, will help the skin to look and feel healthy. By using organic products as much as possible we can reduce the amounts of toxins being absorbed into the body where they can have a knock-on effect on the bladder and other parts of the urinary system.

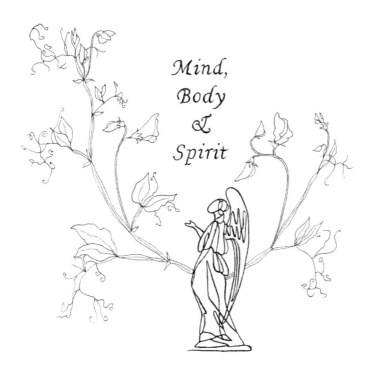

Mind,
Body
&
Spirit

There are many whose bodies are healthy but whose inner being is ill. And, there are also those who suffer some physical disease but whose inner life force is very healthy. All of us will experience some sickness during our lives. That is why it is important to acquire the wisdom to deal with illness properly. [33]

Thoughts and emotions are known to have a direct impact on our state of health, so working on this area can be of great benefit alongside the physical changes and treatments that are undertaken. Although we may not be very aware of it, emotions create chemical reactions within the body and therefore manifest on a physical level. Balancing the psychological, spiritual and physical elements of our lives allows for a holistic approach. This means treating ourselves as a whole – viewing the organs and systems of the body as interconnected – rather than simply applying a treatment that responds to symptoms in each separate area. Eastern cultures tend to address all three aspects – body, mind and spirit – in the process of healing rather than separating the body and mind. The philosophy draws upon the body's ability to heal itself.

There are a number of holistic therapies that encompass the physical, mental and emotional/spiritual to treat the whole body. These include:

• *Homeopathy* – This involves taking minute doses of natural substances derived from plants, animals or minerals in order to stimulate the body's natural healing energy and to restore balance.

• *Bach flower remedies* – These were developed by Dr Edward Bach (1886–1936) and embody the positive aspect of certain conditions in our mental and emotional state (with the negative aspects being viewed as the true cause of illness) to help us to restore health and find happiness.

• *Reiki* – An ancient healing system derived by the Buddhist monk Mikao Usui, which aims to bring about balance and harmony within the body as well as promoting emotional and spiritual well-being. Reiki can also be used as a form of distance healing.

• *Reflexology* - An ancient form of healing which involves massaging the feet – areas of which are believed to reflect an image of organs and systems within the body. These are known as reflex points and pressure is applied to clear blockages and to stimulate the body's immune system to help deal with problems and imbalances.

•   *Acupuncture* – A form of traditional Chinese medicine where needles are applied to particular points along the energy pathways (meridians) in the body to help restore harmony and balance.

•   *Yoga* – This originated in India over 5,000 years ago. Yoga is a Sanskrit word meaning 'union' of mind, body and spirit and the practice, now very popular and well known, involves physical and breathing exercises, relaxation and sometimes meditation.

•   *Tai chi/Qigong* – These involve slow movement exercises – postures, relaxed breathing techniques and a focus of the mind – which enable the free flow of energy (qi) along the meridian pathways. Tai chi is often practised for health reasons but can also be extended to a martial art.

Two years after I had developed the pain in my bladder I embarked on a teacher training course followed a year later by a part-time three year Master's degree in Art Psychotherapy, during which time I was required to be in therapy as part of the training. At the same time I was searching to delve further into the spiritual side of my life in order to enhance the self-healing and I came across a book called *The Buddha in Daily Life: An Introduction to the Buddhism of Nichiren Daishonin* by Richard Causton.

Whilst I was in the middle of reading this book I was invited, by chance, to a Buddhist meeting and since that time I have been practising Nichiren Daishonin's Buddhism. Having been brought up as a Christian, and a regular churchgoer all my life, the transition was not easy but it somehow felt right.

I remember feeling so relieved at those early Buddhist meetings because water is generally provided to everyone rather than tea, coffee or anything alcoholic. It was so refreshing to be able to give the answer 'yes, thank you' and to readily accept what was offered rather than 'no, thank you', which in many circumstances was then followed by some sort of plea or reproach.

A number of workshops were held during the art therapy training. In one of these we were invited to ask someone to draw around us as we lay on a sheet of paper on the floor and then we silently worked on creating an island within the shape of our bodies. Afterwards, as I reflected on what I had produced in the workshop, I realised that I had created a large, red volcano in the pelvic area of my body. I then thought about the burning pain I experienced and the anger I felt in connection with my bladder problem – and how whenever I felt anger, about anything at all, this made the pain in my bladder worse.

One of the principles of Buddhism is the Ten Worlds, or the Ten States of Life, which are ten basic inner states, with Buddhahood being the highest state. Anger is one of the four lower 'life states' and we move between all the states each day from moment to moment.

In Buddhism it is taught that one's mind fluctuates 840 million times a day. The alterations in one's life are, in other words, infinite. One's life is a succession of momentary instances of hot, cold, doubt, delight, sadness and other conditions.[34]

Most of us are likely to find a tendency within ourselves towards the lower life states, but through daily Buddhist practice we have the ability to achieve happiness, as well as to develop feelings of compassion and understanding towards ourselves and others, no matter what obstacles or suffering we are undergoing. We are encouraged to set our own goals and determinations to overcome whatever it is in our lives that we feel we would like to change.

As I carried out the Buddhist chanting, I often envisaged a healing light within my bladder and around that area of my body. At night, before I went to sleep, I would play music that incorporated the soothing sounds of the ocean and envisaged the sea water washing over me and cleansing my whole body. Overall, I felt it was important to see my life beyond a time when it revolved around the pain in my bladder, to feel free from this and restored to good health once again.

It can be confusing to decide which course of action to follow and ongoing treatments can be very expensive. In her book *Nine Ways to Body Wisdom*, Jennifer Harper gives a comprehensive guide to a self-treatment system that anyone can use at home combining nutrition, herbs and spices, exercise, reflexology, acupressure, aromatherapy, flower remedies, affirmations and meditation exercises.

Louise Hay's bestselling book *You Can Heal Your Life* offers a self-healing approach to life and looks at mental patterns that can create dis-ease within the body. It incorporates exercises and ideas to effect changes that are empowering and also encourages the use of daily affirmations.

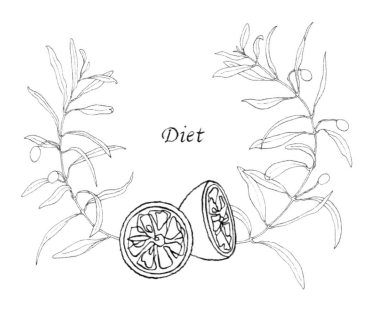

Diet

Each of our bodies is different in terms of what it requires for a healthy diet according to factors such as our constitution, age, lifestyle, current state of health and so on. We may also have developed our own specific reactions to certain foods, producing a variety of negative symptoms and responses, including pain and inflammation in the bladder for those of us who have sensitivity in this area. Managing the best way to cope with this condition may feel like a minefield, but given the correct forms of nourishment the body can begin to heal.

I have already mentioned some of the dangers of eating food that is non-organic – and therefore more likely to contain pesticides and other chemical residues. Choosing fresh, organic ingredients will bring greater benefit to the body as well as helping to cut down on the consumption of processed foods. These include products that are high in saturated fats and sugars such as bread, cakes, biscuits, processed meat and foods made from refined grains. In addition, one of the knock-on effects of eating a high proportion of processed foods is the issue of enzyme deficiency, since some of the enzymes that the body needs are ingested with food. In the absence of these the body needs to use up more of the enzymes that it produces.

Cooking methods are also something to consider. Microwaving significantly decreases the nutritional value of food whilst accelerating its structural disintegration (e.g. it destroys the protein in meat). In addition, microwaved foods make us more susceptible to the cumulative effects of long-term, low-level radiation which can adversely affect the neurological and reproductive systems of the body causing, amongst other things, headaches, sleep disturbance and memory loss. Steaming is a good method of cooking which enables food to retain its vital nutrients and natural flavours. Food that is cooked slowly through baking or stewing is also healthy.

The Slow Food Movement is an organisation with an international profile that was founded by Carlo Petrini in 1986. It campaigns for the move towards 'good, clean and fair' food that tastes good, is produced locally, has a positive impact on the environment and minimum artificial intervention, and for producers to be paid a fair amount for their skill and labour. They have helped set up 'slow food groups' all over the world, which engage with local producers and organise events.

The following is a list of general guidelines for healthy ways of eating:

•   Eat more vegetables and fresh foods – if possible, grow your own.

•   Eat local produce according to the season.

•   Digestion begins in the mouth so chew food properly.

•   Try to eat when relaxed rather than stressed and enjoy the flavours of the food.

•   Drink more water, preferably at room temperature rather than cold (which will cause the stomach to contract and weaken digestion).

•   Avoid or cut down on coffee, tea and alcohol.

•   Try not to eat late in the evening.

•   Eat more alkaline forming foods such as sprouted seeds, fresh fruit and vegetables and brown rice.

•   Eat three or four nutritious meals a day.

•   Use steaming as a way of cooking vegetables to help retain valuable nutrients.

•   Avoid mixing fruit with other foods since it needs to pass through the stomach more quickly.

•   Cut down on or avoid using salt.

•   Eat whole foods rather than those made with refined flours and sugar.

- Cut down on or avoid processed foods.

- Eat more essential fatty acids (see below) and avoid margarine; use olive oil or coconut oil for cooking.

- Use cooking methods other than microwaving and avoid food that has been genetically modified.

- Buy fresh, organic meat as far as possible.

Oils and Fats

Eating the right types of oils and fats can greatly benefit the body – one of the chapters in Sherry Rogers' book *Tired or Toxic?* is 'Are You Due For An Oil Change?'[35]

There are some fats that are essential for the normal functioning of cells in the body known as *essential fatty acids* but processed foods contain *trans-fatty acids*, which have a different molecular structure to non-hydrogenated oils and cause damage to cells in the body. These mainly come in the form of polyunsaturated hydrogenated vegetable oils and margarines. Hydrogenation is a way of extracting oils using high temperatures rather than heavy pressure, as was done in the past, which causes a permanent twisting of the molecular shape. This creates problems including premature aging and a general increase in degenerative disease.

The two main essential fatty acids are omega 3 and omega 6. Omega 6 mainly comes from vegetables and nuts (e.g. safflower, sunflower, borage, sesame). Omega 3 comes from cold water fish (e.g. sardines, mackerel, trout, herring, salmon, tuna), as well as whole grains, beans and seeds (such as linseed and flaxseed). Omega 9 is a naturally occurring fish oil which has a range of benefits including promoting healthy cell membrane structure. The brain is made up of 70% fat, so having enough of the right sort of fats, amongst other things, can make a difference to our brain function, mood and coordination.

Oil that is overheated, particularly in frying, destroys essential fatty acids. Olive oil can stand more heat than the essential fatty acid oils – such as sunflower, linseed, safflower and borage – which should not be used for cooking but can be added to food that has already been cooked.

Organic, cold-pressed oils in glass bottles are best and using these oils over a period of a few months will help to detox the system and revitalise the body. Use cold-pressed olive oil for cooking.

Udo's Choice offers a range of organic omega 3, 6 and 9 oils which are obtained through cold pressing, then filtered and packaged in opaque glass bottles. This oil needs to be kept in the fridge. Dr Udo Erasmus wrote the best-selling book *Fats that Heal, Fats that Kill*, and began his research into nutrition after suffering poisoning from pesticides.

Bio Planete are a French company that make a range of organically certified cold-pressed oils including a blended oil made especially for cooking and frying. Bio Planete virgin oils can usually be found in most health food shops.

The Norwegian company Nordic Naturals make a range of omega supplements including a Complete Omega with omegas 3, 6 and 9 plus vitamin D. They also run a research website (www.omega-research.com) that provides an online resource library looking into the health benefits of essential fatty acids.

Coconut oil can also be used as a cooking oil. The oil contains saturated fats which have antimicrobial properties that can help to deal with harmful bacteria, fungi and parasites affecting the digestive system. It also helps in the absorption of vitamins, minerals and amino acids.

Sprouting Seeds

Sprouting seeds are classed as 'superfoods' since they provide a very high source of protein and contain enzymes which help with digestion and the elimination of toxins, as well as being helpful in the building of new cells. The nutrient content of a seed is dramatically increased by sprouting and these substances are easy for the body to absorb. Another benefit of eating sprouted seeds is that they are alkaline forming foods. Much of what we eat in our diets has an acidifying effect on our bodies which provides a more fertile environment for unwanted bacteria to thrive.

Any type of seed, grain or bean can be sprouted – the 'sprout' is the first growth of the seed where you see the tail appearing from the seed shell. These tails should be about three times the size of the seed itself before eating.

The seeds need to be soaked first (this can be done overnight), then drained and rinsed with water each day until the sprouts appear. Once the sprouted tails have grown long enough, the seeds can finally be put in sunlight to activate the chlorophyll in the plant. Then the sprouted seeds will be ready to eat.

The following is a list of some of the seeds that are commonly used for sprouting:

aduki bean	fenugreek
alfalfa	flax
broccoli	mung bean
chickpea	pumpkin
clover	sesame
fennel	sunflower

It is possible to buy a sprouter kit from health food shops or otherwise a jar can be used with mesh over the top that will hold the seeds in but let the water in and out when rinsing. A.Vogel produces packets of 'biosnacky' seeds for sprouting, some of which come in mixed varieties.

Cress

Cress has good nutritional value and is easy to grow at home on the windowsill by sowing seeds onto damp cotton wool or tissue paper placed on a saucer or other shallow container. The shoots are fast growing and should be ready within about a week to cut and sprinkle on food or to add to salads.

Sea Vegetables (Seaweed)

Seaweeds have been part of the human diet for many centuries but, like many things that were once commonly used and valuable to humans, seaweed has become less valued, although it is still an important part of the diet in Japan.

Seaweeds are extremely rich in minerals, such as potassium, calcium, magnesium and iron and they also contain many vitamins, including vitamin B12. In addition they are beneficial to our health because they absorb toxins and pollutants in the body and help to make the blood more alkaline, thereby helping to counteract acids in the body.

The strong taste of seaweed may take some getting used to but the flavours vary according to the variety. Clearspring sell the following varieties of sea vegetables and have recipes and information on each type on their website: nori, arame, dulse, kombu, wakame, hijiki and agar flakes.

I mainly use wakame, which has thin leaves and a mild flavour, and hijiki which is also thin-leaved and helps to give the Japanese their beautiful, shiny hair. Kombu is broad-leaved and has a stronger flavour and this can be added to stocks and soups.

Carob

Carob comes from an evergreen tree that is native to the Mediterranean and Middle East and has been cultivated for over 4,000 years. It produces edible seed pods that are about 20 cm long. Carob makes a good chocolate substitute as it contains 40% natural sugar but is lower in fat and is a rich source of calcium and potassium, as well as containing small amounts of iron and some B vitamins.

Carob powder is made from the ground bean and can be used as an alternative to drinking chocolate and cocoa powder. I have found that some carob powders have a better taste than others since they can sometimes have a slightly burnt flavour. Hambleden Herbs produce a powder that meets Soil Association organic standards and is the one that I prefer.

Eating According to Blood Type

After hearing about a diet based on eating foods according to your blood type, I sought out *Eat Right 4 Your Type* by Dr Peter D'Adamo. He has carried out research in this area and it may be something to consider when planning a healthy diet.

Type 'O' is the most common blood type and these people were originally hunter-gatherers living on meat, fish, fruit but no grains or dairy products. Those with blood type 'A' descended from farmers and ate more grain produce and less meat. Type 'B' evolved from a mingling of tribes and can eat more freely from most types of foods, and those with type 'AB', the rarest blood group, can eat a combination of diets for types 'A' and 'B'.

Warming and Cooling Foods

Many diets recommend eating raw foods as these are often considered to be more healthy, but in Traditional

Chinese Medicine foods are deemed to have different properties – some are warming and raise our metabolic rate and others are cooling and lower it. It is generally best to eat more raw, or cooling, foods in the summer months or else balance out with some warming foods. These are cooked foods, particularly food that has been cooked slowly such as in a bake or a stew. Ginger is a spice with warming properties and can be added to food when cooking. Each of us is different and we need to find a diet that suits us and creates balance within our bodies, but the seasons and climate also can be used as a gauge by which we can plan our diet with an aim to eat food that is appropriate for the time of year.

Lemon Detox Diet (Natural Tree Syrup)

This is a diet based on a cleansing programme developed by the naturopath Stanley Burroughs in 1941. It has been refined in the creation of Madal Bal Natural Tree Syrup, a Swiss product made up of a combination of Southeast Asian palm syrups and grade C+ Canadian maple syrup (which is rich in mineral content and is not the same as regular maple syrup). The syrup is mixed with lemon juice, cayenne pepper and water to prepare a drink that can be taken over a period of a few days without food, known as the 'total detox' programme, or else as a substitute for one or two meals per day over a period of time. This is known as the 'relaxed diet'.

The main purpose is to cleanse the body of accumulated toxins from artificial additives and other chemicals in foods as well as those in our environment. Some of the benefits are: an increase in energy, healthier hair and nails, clearer skin and eyes and improved digestion.

Natural Tree Syrup can be found in many health food shops. A leaflet comes with the product explaining its background and benefits and there is also a book called *The Lemon Detox Diet: Rejuvenation Sensation* by Dr K. A. Beyer.

I tried this diet for three days having never fasted before and found it fairly difficult, but there are many testimonials from people who have carried out the 'total detox' programme and felt great benefit. Since then I have occasionally done the relaxed diet for a day at a time to help cleanse my system.

Snacks

One of the difficulties of being on a healthy diet can be what to eat if you feel the need for something in-between meals. Most snack foods come in a packet, together with additives and often many of the other things that one is trying to avoid, especially when carrying out an anti-candida programme and sugar is top of the list.

Sunflower seeds are remarkably filling as well as being a good source of omega 6 and they can be bought in a variety of shops.

Clearspring make an assortment of *rice cakes* and *crackers* in different shapes and sizes, which are tasty and filling and can be bought in many health food shops or via the internet.

Oatcakes come in a range of makes and varieties and are another food that can be eaten as a snack on their own. Some contain wheat and occasionally sugar so it is best to check on the packet before buying.

Avocado pears are nutritious and filling and one sliced in half and eaten with either an omega oil or olive oil poured into the hollow left by the large seed provides a healthy and tasty snack.

Rice noodles are quick and easy to cook. I sometimes add a little salt to the water and an egg, which poaches whilst the noodles are cooking. Once out of the pan I then add some omega or olive oil and cress or salad leaves.

Bananas are generally known to be a filling fruit but it is best to eat organic.

Carob drink made with 1–2 teaspoons of carob powder and heated *Oatly* or *Vanilla Rice Dream* is a favourite of mine and a good alternative to hot chocolate.

Sushi makes a very tasty snack and is not too difficult to make once you have the right ingredients. Clearspring sell sushi rice, nori (edible roasted seaweed sheets) and the mats for rolling sushi (recipes are also available on their website – www.clearspring.co.uk).

Breakfast

Breakfast is generally a healthy and uncomplicated meal giving us energy at the start of the day, but it is the one most likely to be missed. What we eat for breakfast can form an important part of our daily intake of essential nutrients. *Milk* – If avoiding milk there are now many dairy-free alternatives such as *soya milk*, *Oatly* made from pure oats and *Rice Dream* made from rice, which comes in different varieties. These products are organic and do not contain added sugars.

Cereal – Many cereals contain sugar but it is now easier to find cereals that are sugar-free and wheat-free. Doves Farm makes a range of organic cereals including gluten- and sugar-free cornflakes.

Porridge – Choose between ground or rolled oats for making porridge, and a milk alternative can be used if adding milk with the water.

Eggs – Fried, poached or scrambled eggs (made with a milk alternative) can be eaten with oat or rice cakes as an alternative to bread.

Tiffin Box Lunches

Maintaining a healthy diet when away from home for any reason, such as being at work all day, can be extremely difficult if certain foods, particularly bread and yeast, need to be avoided. But a well-sealed tiffin box may be filled with whatever you like, including leftovers. Tiffin is an Anglo-Indian word meaning 'snack' which originated in Southern India at a time when British workers were not accustomed to the spicy Indian food so they arranged for a special lunch to be delivered to them at work. The lunch boxes, known as a *dabba*, were delivered by dabawallahs, and this trade has since passed through generations of families who came from the Deccan Plateau, near Mumbai, and continues to be in use today.

Sometimes I get asked whether the food in it is kept hot, perhaps because one might expect to find hot food inside a metal tin. All types of cooked food can be eaten cold, such as rice, potatoes, vegetables and pasta as well as cooked meats. It is the combination of ingredients and flavours and how the food was cooked and prepared that is important. Extra food can be cooked when preparing an evening meal and the leftovers eaten for lunch.

Stainless steel tiffin boxes can be bought either online or through shops that sell general household goods. My box is approximately 14 cm in diameter and 6 cm deep and is a single tin, although tiffin carriers can also come in layers of three or four. The following is a handful of ideas for lunches that can be put together and transported in a container such as a tiffin box:

Chicken

Avocado

Rice or brown rice pasta

Sunflower seeds

Watercress/Nasturtium flowers

Tomatoes

Udo's Choice oil

Mackerel

Roast sweet potato slices

French beans

Parsley

Pine kernels

Udo's Choice oil

Tofu burger

Rice or brown rice pasta

Sprouted seeds

Lettuce

Basil

Grated carrot

Avocado

A little olive oil

Organic ham

Roast fennel

Brown rice with coriander

Cress

Steamed carrots

Mange tout

Parsley

Safflower oil

Sardines

Steamed new potatoes

Fried or baked courgette

Chives/Parsley

Steamed broccoli

Sprouted seeds

Tomatoes

Chicken

Roast peppers

Steamed potatoes

Steamed carrots and beans

Roast aubergine

Sunflower seeds

Udo's Choice oil

Organic bacon

Brown or wild rice

Roasted sweet potatoes

Chives

Steamed carrot, broccoli and courgette

Sprouted seeds

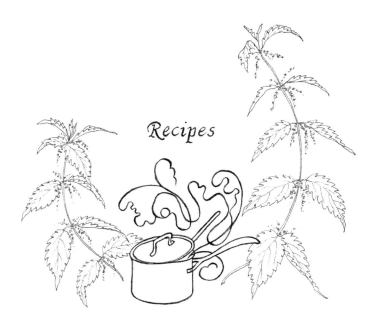

Recipes

Breakfast

Porridge with Cinnamon

There are many different ways of cooking this traditional Scottish dish, and possibly a greater variety of oats to choose from nowadays to make it with. I prefer to use medium organic rolled oats. A spoonful of honey can be added at the end and sometimes I add a small amount of grated ginger during the cooking process to make a warming breakfast in the winter. Cinnamon has a variety of health benefits as it is a source of manganese, calcium and iron and, amongst other things, it can be helpful against yeast infections.

rolled oats

water

½ teaspoon of cinnamon

Oatly

Soak the oats in water overnight. Add double the quantity of water, along with the cinnamon. Cook over a low heat and keep stirring every so often adding more water if necessary. Serve with Oatly or almond milk.

Soups

Stocks for making soups

I find that a good homemade stock, rather than one prepared from stock cubes, makes a great difference to the tastiness of a soup and it is healthier too. Most stock cubes contain sugar, yeast extract and sometimes monosodium glutamate.

Chicken: To make chicken stock either boil a whole chicken and then take the meat off the bone, or use the carcass of a roasted chicken once all the meat has been removed. Add a peeled potato, an onion, carrots, two cloves of garlic and a good handful of herbs, such as sage, marjoram, thyme and tarragon, to a large pan and fill nearly to the top with water. Add some seaweed, such as kombu, arame, dulse or hijiki, to the pot, as these provide additional sources of vitamins and minerals. Then bring to the boil and simmer for about an hour. Strain the liquid into a ceramic bowl. Leave to go cold and then put in the fridge overnight so that if there is any fat it will set on the top. This fat can be removed with a spoon and used for cooking separately in other recipes.

Bacon Lardons: This is something that I have recently started to use for making stock since I can buy small packets of smoked bacon lardons quite cheaply at my local farmers' market. I think they add a particularly good flavour to winter soups. Lardons are thick pieces of chopped bacon but it is also possible to use thickly cut bacon rashers as an alternative. Boil up the lardons with a potato, carrot, onion, three bay leaves, two cloves of garlic, rosemary, sage and a sprinkling of seaweed. Strain the liquid into a bowl and then, once cooled, remove the fat from the bacon chunks and break them up into smaller pieces. Set aside to add to soups or stews.

Butternut Squash and Parsnip Soup

1 butternut squash

2 parsnips

1 potato

1 large onion

a small handful of fresh sage

1 clove of garlic

arame seaweed

750 ml–1 litre of chicken or other stock

butter or olive oil

1 teaspoon of chopped parsley

Chop the onion and fry it in a little butter or olive oil and a couple of tablespoons of the chicken stock for about ten minutes with the pan lid on. Keep stirring the onion every so often so it does not stick to the bottom of the pan. Add the chopped sage and garlic, stir and fry for a minute or two. Peel and chop the squash, parsnips and potato. Add these to the pan with a small sprinkling of arame seaweed and then pour over the chicken stock. Add enough water to cover the vegetables, bring to the boil and cook for about thirty minutes or until all the vegetables are soft. Take off the heat, either mash or blend and add salt and pepper to taste. Serve with a sprinkling of chopped parsley.

Carrot, Leek and Sweet Potato Soup with Bacon

3 medium carrots

1 large leek

1 large sweet potato

1 onion

1 clove of garlic

arame seaweed

a handful of chopped herbs

750 ml–1 litre of stock made using bacon lardons

cooked bacon pieces

water

a little butter or olive oil

Chop the onion and fry it in a little butter or olive oil and a couple of tablespoons of the stock for about ten minutes with the pan lid on. Keep stirring the onion every so often so it does not stick to the bottom of the pan. Add the chopped herbs and garlic, stir and fry for a minute or two. Peel and chop the carrots, leek and sweet potato and add to the pan with a small sprinkling of arame seaweed and then pour over the stock. Add enough water to cover the vegetables, bring to the boil and cook for about thirty minutes or until all the vegetables are soft. Take off the heat, either mash or blend the soup and add the cooked bacon pieces. Add salt and pepper to taste.

Nettle Soup

Nettles have been eaten for centuries and are of high nutritional value since they are a good source of minerals, including iron, magnesium and vitamins. It is best to pick the young leaves from the tops of the nettle plants in spring, protecting your hands with gloves so as not to get stung.

bunch of hand-picked nettle tops

1 onion

2 potatoes

1 litre of stock

fresh parsley

Chop the onion and fry it in a little butter or olive oil and a couple of tablespoons of the stock for about ten minutes with the pan lid on. Peel and chop the potatoes and cook in the stock with the lid on for about ten minutes or until soft. Add the washed nettle tops and some fresh parsley and simmer for five to ten minutes. Liquidise the soup and add salt and pepper to taste.

Salads

Omega oils are a healthy alternative to traditional salad dressings and adding them to salads is the best way to eat the oil since it cannot be heated.

Watercress, Avocado and Pine Kernel Salad with Nasturtium Flowers

Watercress is full of nutrients and is sometimes described as a 'superfood'. Nasturtiums come from the same plant family as watercress and are easy to grow in the garden, producing a profusion of colourful flowers throughout the summer. Both watercress and nasturtiums have a peppery flavour.

pine kernels

watercress

nasturtium flowers

1 avocado pear

oil or dressing

Bake the pine kernels in the oven until they turn golden. Peel and slice the avocado pear and place on a bed of watercress. Sprinkle over the pine kernels and place the nasturtium flowers on the top. Drizzle over a dressing of your choice.

Celeriac, Carrot and Sprouted Seeds

Celeriac is a type of celery that is grown for its bulbous root. It has a similar flavour to the stalk celery that is commonly available. It has a long growing season and the root of the plant will be ready for eating from about October and on throughout the winter. It can be eaten either raw or cooked.

1 celeriac root

2 medium carrots

1 tablespoon of sprouted seeds

oil or dressing

Cut away the outer layer from the celeriac and grate the peeled root. Peel and grate the carrots and mix with the celeriac and sprouted seeds. Mix in some oil or dressing.

Fennel, Cress, Tomato and Fresh Mint

Florence fennel has been cultivated in the Mediterranean and Asia for centuries and is a popular vegetable in Italy but, so far, I have had no success at growing it myself since it is very sensitive to having the right conditions to reach maturity. The bulb of the plant has a mild aniseed flavour and can be eaten either raw in salads or cooked.

1 fennel bulb

cress

tomatoes

fresh mint leaves

Cut off the top of the fennel bulb, slice in half and then cut out the hard core at the base of the bulb. Slice the remainder of the bulb as finely as possible and put into a bowl with the cress, sliced tomatoes and chopped mint leaves. Mix with a little oil or dressing.

Main Dishes

I have not included salt and pepper in the recipes below but these can be added according to your taste.

Chicken with Coriander and Lime

4 chicken thighs

1 onion

1 clove of garlic

1 tablespoon of chopped fresh coriander

juice of ½ a lime

chopped fresh root ginger

2 potatoes

water or vegetable stock

oil for cooking

Use a casserole pot and fry the onion in the oil until it is soft and then put to one side. Fry the pieces of chicken until browned on each side. Add the cooked onion, garlic, coriander, lime juice, peeled and chopped potato and chopped ginger. Cover with water or vegetable stock, place the lid on the top and cook in an oven at 180°C/365°F for fifty minutes. Serve with rice or steamed new potatoes and vegetables.

Steamed Chicken with Lemon Thyme

Fish can also be cooked in the same way for this recipe.

chicken breasts

juice of ½ lemon

lemon thyme

olive oil

Tear off a piece of parchment paper one and a half times the length of each chicken breast and at least three times the width. Place a chicken breast in the centre of each piece and add some lemon thyme and a little lemon juice and olive oil. Pull up the sides of the paper and fold over twice at the top and then fold in the ends so that the juices remain in the parcel. Place the chicken parcel in a steamer with the water already boiling and steam for about twenty minutes, or until the chicken is cooked through. Serve with new potatoes and green vegetables.

Salmon Steaks with Ginger

This is very quick and easy to cook and can be served with steamed potatoes and green vegetables, such as French beans or chard.

salmon steaks

fresh root ginger

oil for cooking

Put the salmon steaks into an ovenproof dish and grate some of the root ginger onto the top of each one. Pour over a little oil and cook uncovered in an oven at 180°C/365°F for about fifteen minutes.

Sausage and Mash

6 organic sausages

2 onions

1 courgette

thyme

sage

potato

celeriac

Oatly

Chop the onion and put it in an ovenproof dish. Place the sausages on top. Cut the top off the courgette and then slice it in half lengthways and then cut each half in two lengthways and place the courgette in-between the sausages. Sprinkle on some chopped sage leaves and thyme and add a drizzle of olive oil over the top. Bake in an oven at 180°C/365°F for forty minutes, turning the sausages halfway through.

For the mash, peel and chop the potatoes and remove the outer skin from the celeriac root. Chop the celeriac root into cubes and steam with the potatoes until they are soft. Put them into a warm dish or pan and mash with a little Oatly as required.

Slow Cooked Beef Brisket

I buy brisket from my local farmers' market, already taken off the bone and rolled. Brisket is the cut of beef from the breast of the animal and it tends to be less expensive than other cuts since it is fairly tough and therefore needs to be cooked slowly. Slow cookers are the perfect way to do this and using this method requires little effort once the food has been prepared.

A slow cooker is an electric appliance, either round or oval in shape, which only heats up to moderate temperatures, so you don't have to worry about timing as the food cannot overcook, although some slow cookers do come with automatic timers. Slow cookers are also good for casseroles or cooking a whole chicken or pheasant together with vegetables to create food that is tender and flavoursome.

beef brisket

2 onions or half a dozen shallots

2 potatoes

1 parsnip

2 carrots

2 bay leaves

rosemary

thyme

water

red wine (optional)

brown rice flour

Peel and chop the vegetables. Put some of the vegetables into the slow cooker and then place the brisket in the centre. Add the rest of the vegetables and the herbs all around the meat. Pour in enough water and the wine (if using) to almost cover the meat and vegetables and leave for several hours (I leave mine for the whole day) on a low heat setting to cook. Remove the beef and use a cup to take out a cupful of juice. Add two tablespoons of brown rice flour to the cup and mix together. Spoon this back into the slow cooker and stir it in to thicken the juice. Turn up the heat and leave to cook for a little longer.

It always surprises me that vegetables can take longer to cook than meat, but using this method of cooking I have noticed that the vegetables can sometimes do with a little more cooking time. Slice the meat and serve it together with the vegetables and juice.

Rice Pasta with Bacon and Basil

Doves Farm make penne from organic brown rice, which is a good alternative to products made with wheat and it is just as quick and easy to cook.

brown rice penne pasta

bacon

fresh basil

olive or omega oil

Either grill or cook the bacon in the oven. Then cut the bacon into small pieces (scissors can be the easiest method for doing this). Bring a pan of water to the boil. Add the required amount of pasta and cook for 5–7 minutes. Add the bacon, fresh basil and a little olive or omega oil.

Vegetables

Baked Beetroot

Beetroot tends to grow well on my allotment, therefore I try to sow as much of it as possible in the spring so that I can harvest it right through until the winter. The leaves can also be eaten like spinach, only needing a short cooking time (I usually do this in a steamer).

beetroot

1 clove of garlic

thyme

olive oil

Peel and dice the beetroot. Put it into a heavy ovenproof dish with a lid. Add a little olive oil, some fresh thyme and the peeled and chopped garlic. Put on the lid and bake in an oven at 180°C/365°F for forty minutes. If you do not have a heavy ovenproof dish line the dish with parchment paper and wrap this over the beetroot before putting the lid on to bake.

Roast Aubergine

As a member of the nightshade family the aubergine is closely related to the potato and tomato, although it is a tropical and sub-tropical plant native to India and needs high temperatures to produce fruits. The white, oval-shaped fruits of some eighteenth century varieties resembled goose eggs, which is why they are also known as eggplants in some parts of the world.

1 medium or large aubergine

1 clove of garlic

olive oil

Cut the top off the aubergine to remove the remainder of the stem. Then cut the fruit in half lengthways to reveal the flesh inside. Score this with a knife to create a criss-cross pattern, cutting deeply but avoiding slicing through the skin beneath. Put the two halves open side up in an ovenproof dish. Crush the clove of garlic and spread this over the aubergine halves, pressing down so that the garlic gets pushed into the cuts in the flesh. Pour some olive oil onto each half. Bake in an oven at 180°C/365°F for twenty-five minutes. Turn over and bake for a further ten minutes, adding more oil if necessary.

Rice with Tomato and Herbs

This is a simple recipe but you can add other ingredients, such as finely chopped fresh ginger and a variety of herbs for more taste. Adding a sprinkling of seaweed provides an easy way for the body to take in important minerals whilst having little effect on the taste of the dish. I also sometimes chop a courgette into segments and layer the pieces on the top so that they cook at the same time with the rice, but end up as a separate layer once the rice is cooked. The same can be done with other green vegetables, such as kale, chard or purple sprouting broccoli. It is best to use a heavy bottomed pan for this recipe.

1 cupful of rice (wholegrain brown rice is less starchy and more nutritious than white rice)

1 onion

1 chopped clove of garlic

hijiki or arame seaweed

water or stock

1 tablespoon of coriander seeds (optional)

1 cm cube of fresh ginger finely chopped (optional)

½ tin of plum peeled tomatoes or 1 chopped beef tomato

cooking oil

Chop the onion and fry it in the oil until it becomes soft. Add the rice and stir it into the onion before adding the tomatoes. Cook for a couple of minutes and stir so that it doesn't stick to the bottom of the pan. Add the chopped garlic, coriander seeds and ginger and two cupfuls of water or one cupful of water and one cupful of stock. Sprinkle the seaweed on the top, give the ingredients a stir and put the lid on the pan, bring to the boil and then simmer until all the water has been absorbed.

Puddings and Biscuits

All forms of sugar should be avoided, as well as wheat, when carrying out an anti-candida diet, so I have just included three sweet recipes – the diet is not forever. I now try to use rice flour rather than wheat flour as much as possible for baking and other recipes.

Baked Bananas with Honey

bananas

zest of half a lemon

honey

cinnamon

Peel and slice the bananas lengthways and place the two pieces side by side in the centre of a piece of parchment paper big enough to make into a parcel. Sprinkle on some lemon zest, cinnamon and add a teaspoon of honey. Fold the parchment over at the top and at both ends and then put into an ovenproof dish. Cook in the oven at 180°C/365°F for ten to fifteen minutes.

Apple with Bread Topping

This is an adapted version of a recipe that I saw on television which used breadcrumbs as an alternative topping for an apple crumble. The second time I made it I cut up the bread into small chunks rather than making breadcrumbs and I found that I liked this better, but either method can be used for the topping.

3 cooking apples

120 g (4 oz) of butter

3 tablespoons of soft brown sugar

stem ginger

zest of half a lemon

water

1 small wholemeal loaf (unsliced)

Peel and core the apples and then cut into slices. Arrange these in layers in an ovenproof dish. Add two tablespoons of water, sprinkle over the lemon zest and a little of the sugar. Slice half a piece of stem ginger and tuck in amongst the apple and then pour over a little syrup from the jar of stem ginger. Melt the butter in a saucepan and then dissolve the remaining sugar in the butter. Cut the bread into lots of small chunks (you may not need to use the whole loaf) and mix this into the butter and sugar. Spread the bread mixture over the top of the apple and bake in the oven at 180°C/365°F for thirty-five minutes.

Orange and Almond Biscuits

180 g (6 oz) of butter

90 g (3 oz) of caster sugar

150 g (5 oz) of plain flour

50 g (2 oz) of brown rice flour

50 g (2 oz) of ground almonds

flaked almonds for decoration

Mix all the ingredients together in a bowl to form a soft dough and then roll it into a ball. Add a little more rice flour if the mixture is too sticky or a little more butter if it will not form a dough. Sprinkle some flour onto a flat surface and roll out the dough. Use a biscuit cutter to cut the biscuit rounds, place them on a greased baking tray and put a flaked almond in the centre of each one. Bake in the oven at 180°C/365°F for fifteen minutes, or until the biscuits have cooked to a golden colour on top.

Notes

1. Ikeda, D. (1999) *Humanism and the Art of Medicine.* SGI Malaysia, p. 5.

2. See   http://www.nhs.uk/conditions/urinary-tract-infection-adults/Pages/Introduction.aspx (accessed 8 December 2010).

3. Gillespie, L. (1996) *You Don't Have to Live with Cystitis.* Avon Books, p. 55.

4. Ibid., p. 63.

5. Ibid., p. 103

6. Ibid., p. 68.

7. *The Sunday Times*, Style Magazine, 20 August 2000, p.39

8. Martin Crook quoted in Martin, S. (1998) *The Natural Way: Candida.* Element, p. xi.

9. Chaitow, L. (1996) *Candida Albicans: The Non-Drug Approach to the Treatment of Candida Infection –*

The Proliferation of a Parasite Yeast That Lives Inside All of Us. Thorsons, p. 75.

10. Trenev, N. (1998) *Probiotics: Nature's Internal Healers – Your Body's First Line of Defense against Most Common Diseases.* Avery Publishing, p. ix.

11. Ibid., p.157.

12. Martin, *The Natural Way: Candida*, p. 56

13. Chaitow, *Candida Albicans,* p. 75.

14. Bartnett, B. (2001) *Urine-Therapy: It May Save Your Life!* Lifestyle Institute, p. 2.

15. Ibid., p. 1.

16. Ibid., p. 17.

17. Sharp, S. *Miraculous Messages from Water: How water reflects our consciousness.* www.wellnessgoods.com/messages.asp (accessed 8 December 2010).

18. Emoto, M. (2001) The Hidden Messages in Water. Beyond Words Publishing, p. 68.

19. Price, B. (1983) *A Friends of the Earth Guide to Pollution.* Maurice Temple Smith, p. 19.

20. Ibid., p. 18.

21. Rogers, S. H. (1998) *Tired or Toxic? A Blueprint for Health.* Prestige Publishers, p. 103.

22. Price, *Friends of the Earth*, p. 19.

23. See http://www.holisticdentalcentre.co.uk/ mercury free.html. (accessed 8 December 2010)

24.   Simone, C. M. (2000) *Along the Healing Path: Recovering from Interstitial Cystitis.*__Morris Publishing, p. 121.

25.   Grigson, S. and Black, W. (2001) *Organic: A New Way of Eating*, Headline, p. 40.

26.   See http://www.pan-uk.org/publications/other (accessed 8 December 2010).

27.   Brostoff, J. and Gamlin, L. (1989) *The Complete Guide to Food Allergy and Intolerance,* Bloomsbury. p.180.

28.   Harley, K. (2009, July 21) Available at www.environmentalhealthnews.org/ehs/newscien ce/children-are-more-vulnerable-to-pesticides-until-age-7. (accessed 8 December 2010).

29.   Brostoff and Gamlin, *The Complete Guide to Food Allergy and Intolerance,* p. 184.

30.   Wohl, A. (1984) *Endangered Lives: Public Health in Victorian Britain.* Methuen, p. 24.

31.   See http://ww2.defra.gov.uk/environment/quality/air/ air-quality. *Air Quality.* (accessed 25 January 2011).

32.   Harper, J. (2000) *Nine Ways to Body Wisdom: Blending Natural Therapies to Nourish Body, Emotions and Soul.* Thorsons, p. 210.

33.   Ikeda, *Art of Medicine*, p. 9.

34.   Causton, R. (1995) *The Buddha in Daily Life: An Introduction to the Buddhism of Nichiren Daishonin.* Rider, p. 38.

35.   Rogers, *Tired or Toxic?*, p. 205.

Useful Addresses and Websites

Networks and Organisations

British Society for Mercury Free Dentistry
The Weathervane
22A Moorend Park Road
Cheltenham
Gloucestershire GL5 30JY
Tel: +44 (0)1242 226 918
www.mercuryfreedentistry.org.uk

The Cystitis and Overactive Bladder (COB) Association
Kings Court
17 School Road

Hall Green

Birmingham B28 8JG

Tel: +44 (0)121 702 0820

www.cobfoundation.org

National Institute of Medical Herbalists

Elm House

54 Mary Arches Street

Exeter EX4 3BA

Tel: +44 (0)1392 426022

www.nimh.org.uk

The Organic Food Directory – Food, Wine and Lifestyle

This website provides information on all aspects of organic living, from food and local organic markets to organic clothing and holidays.

www.organicliving.ukf.net

Pesticide Action Network (PAN) UK

A non-profit organisation working nationally and internationally with individuals concerned with health and the environment. It promotes safer alternatives to pesticides, the production of healthy food and sustainable farming. The website gives information on the best and worst foods for pesticide residues.

Development House

56–64 Leonard Street

London EC2A 4LT

Tel: +44 (0)207 065 0905

www.pan-uk.org

Soka Gakkai International (SGI) UK

The UK arm of the SGI, a Buddhist Society which is established in 192 countries around the world.

Taplow Court

Taplow

Berkshire SL6 0ER

Tel: +44 (0)1628 773163

www.sgi-uk.org

Slow Food UK

Organises projects and events around the UK.

6 Neal's Yard

Covent Garden

London WC2H 9DP

Tel: +44 (0)207 099 1132

www.slowfood.org.uk

Supplements and Health Products

A.Vogel Herbal Remedies

Provides information on a range of fresh herbal tinctures manufactured in Switzerland where the company was founded by the Swiss naturopath Alfred Vogel. Produced and distributed by Bioforce (UK) Ltd.

Tel: +44 (0)1294 277 344

www.avogel.co.uk

Higher Nature

Vitamin, mineral and other healthcare products.

Burwash Common

East Sussex TN19 7LX

Tel: +44 (0)1435 883 484

www.highernature.co.uk

Nordic Naturals

Norwegian company producing omega oils and supplements. The website provides a link to find a store that sells their products near you.

www.nordicnaturals.com

ParaSend

Website selling French beauty and healthcare products including the Arkopharma range.

Tel: +44 (0)3899 10202

www.parasend.com

Revital

Stores in London and parts of the UK selling health foods, supplements, books, etc.

Tel: +44 (0)870 366 5729

www.revital.co.uk

Solgar

Online store for Solgar vitamin and mineral supplements.

www.solgar.co.uk

Sweet Cures

Supply Waterfall D-Mannose and other supplements that provide natural bladder and urinary tract support.

Unit 7

Pyramid Court

Rosetta Way

York YO65 5NB

Tel: 44 (0)1904 789 559

www.waterfall-d-mannose.com

Foods and Other Products for Healthy Living

Avalon Organics

Cosmetic and body care products made with selected organic ingredients and without the use of harmful chemicals.

www.avalonorganics.com

BigGreenSmile.com

Website selling a wide range of natural and eco-friendly products.

Tel: 0845 230 2365 (+44 17535 88405 from outside the UK)

www.biggreensmile.com

Bio Planete

Website for producers of Bio Planete organic oils.

www.bioplanete.com

Bio-Life International Ltd

Offers a range of skincare and other products for allergy sufferers.

Tel: +44 (0)1608 686 626

www.bio-life.co.uk

Clearspring Ltd

Produce organic and traditional food including sea vegetables. Also gives recipes on website.

19a Acton Park Estate

London W3 7QE

Tel: +44 (0)208 749 1781

www.clearspring.co.uk

Doves Farm Foods Ltd

Organic gluten-free flour specialists offering a range of organic, gluten-free products.

Salisbury Road

Hungerford

Berkshire RG17 0RF

Tel: +44 (0)1488 684 880

www.dovesfarm.co.uk

Dr. Hauschka

Organic skincare products.

Tel: +44 (0)1386 791 022

www.drhauschka.co.uk

Forever Living

Health and skincare products based on *Aloe vera*.

Tel: 0844 875 4050

www.foreverliving.com

The Green People Company Ltd

Specialises in organic body care products.

Pondtail Farm

Coolham Road

West Grinstead

West Sussex RH13 8LN

Tel: +44 (0)1403 740350

www.greenpeople.co.uk

Greens Water Systems

Company selling water products including distillers and drinking water systems.

Longacre Business Park

Westminster Road

North Hykeham

Lincoln LN6 3QH

Tel: +44 (0)1522 509 383

www.water-systems.co.uk

Hambledon Herbs

Organic, soil association certified products including teas, infusions, herbs, spices and herbal remedies. Also have recipes on website.

Rushall Organic Farm

Devizes Road

Rushall

Wiltshire SN9 6ET

Tel: +44 (0)1980 630 721

www.hambledenherbs.co.uk

The Healthy House Ltd

Mail order business selling a wide range of products for allergy sufferers and those with chemical sensitivities.

The Old Co-op

Lower Street

Ruscombe

Stroud

Gloucestershire GL6 6BU

Tel: 0845 450 5950 (+44 (0)1453 752 216 from outside the UK)

www.thehealthyhouse.co.uk

Neal's Yard Remedies

Company which makes and sells a range of organic health and beauty products, including a wide range of dried herbs.

NYR Direct

Peacemarsh

Gillingham

Dorset SP8 4EU

Tel: 0845 262 3145

www.nealsyardremedies.com

Oatly

A range of products made from oats. Also gives recipes on website.

www.oatly.com

Further Reading

BARTNETT, B. (2001) *Urine-Therapy: It May Save Your Life!* Lifestyle Institute.

BEYER, K. A. (2006) *The Lemon Detox Diet: Rejuvenation Sensation*. PNP Ltd.

BROSTOFF, J. and GAMLIN, L. (1989) *The Complete Guide to Food Allergy and Intolerance.* Bloomsbury.

CAUSTON, R. (1995) *The Buddha in Daily Life: An Introduction to the Buddhism of Nichiren Daishonin.* Rider.

CHAITOW, L. (1996) *Candida Albicans: The Non-Drug Approach to the Treatment of Candida Infection – The Proliferation of a Parasite Yeast that Lives Inside All of Us.* Thorsons.

D'ADAMO, P. (1996) *Eat Right 4 Your Type.* G.P. Putham's Sons.

EMOTO, M. (2005) *The Hidden Messages in Water*. Simon & Schuster.

ERASMUS, U. (1999) *Fats that Heal, Fats that Kill.* Alive Books.

GILLESPIE, L. (1996) *You Don't Have to Live with Cystitis.* Avon Books.

HARPER, J. (2000) *Nine Ways to Body Wisdom: Blending Natural Therapies to Nourish Body, Emotions and Soul.* Thorsons.

HARVEY, G. (1998) *The Killing of the Countryside.* Vintage.

HAY, L. (1984) *You Can Heal Your Life.* Hay House Publishing.

JEFFERS, S. (2007) *Feel the Fear and Do It Anyway.* Vermilion.

LEVENSON, F. (2000) *Menace in the Mouth.* What Doctors Don't Tell You Ltd.

ROGERS, S. H. (1998) *Tired or Toxic? A Blueprint for Health.* Prestige Publishers.

SIMONE, C. M. (2000) *Along the Healing Path: Recovering from Interstitial Cystitis.* Morris Publishing.

TRENEV, N. (1998) *Probiotics: Nature's Internal Healers – Your Body's First Line of Defense against Most Common Diseases.* Avery Publishing.

WILLIAMS, X. (1998) *Overcoming Candida: The Ultimate Cookery Guide.* Element Books.

WOLVERTON, B. C. (1997) *How to Grow Fresh Air: 50 Houseplants that Purify Your Home or Office.* Penguin.